100&
HEALTHY

More Praise for 100 & Healthy

"Shaffer Fox has provided doctors and the public alike with the only comprehensive book about primary Georgian plant medicines—herbs which have been shown to prevent, slow the progression of, and treat nearly every major degenerative disease. This is exhaustively documented information previously unknown to the West. Mr. Fox not only details all the research to date, he also outlines the criteria for finding high quality products which contain the correct plant materials. Anyone seriously interested in living a longer and healthier life should read *100 & Healthy!*"

– Carolyn DeMarco, M.D.

"This book accurately separates fact from fiction. An amazing intellectual journey into the land of my birth—the land of my grandfather, who lived to be 113 years old. The longevity nutrients described in this book are real, and have been studied within Georgian scientific circles for decades."

– Zakir Ramazanov, Ph.D., former Chief of the Department of Biotechnology of the Soviet Academy of Sciences

"This book is interesting, extremely well-researched and well-written, and very enlightening. It primarily focuses on four unique nutritional substances, each of which I have tested, and each of which are of the highest quality—a level of quality which far exceeds all norms of the nutritional products industry."

– Jeff Levin, R.N.C.

"A whole library in itself! This work can be easily read and studied in depth. It expands on every detail being exposed, and it leaves no stones unturned. What a feat!"

– Marjorie Smith, M.D.

"The author effectively connects the dots from traditional Georgian dietary lifestyle and folk medicines to their effects on preventing and treating disease (thereby extending healthy longevity) to their validation by modern science. The sheer artistry of Georgian tradition and today's science become one in this remarkable book."
— Gerhard Wolfgang Fuchs, Ph.D.

"Mr. Fox writes to us in the language of the natural and social sciences—and he does so in a way that can be understood by everyone. He does not delve into the metaphysical or even the existential; instead he deals with cold, hard facts, and through his exposition of those facts we can form our own judgments. *100 & Healthy* is a marvelous, thought-provoking work!"
— Iago Kachkachishvili, Ph.D., Tblisi State University, Republic of Georgia

"Shaffer Fox zeroes in on the historical bases of Georgian longevity. Extremely interesting, well-researched, and well-documented."
— Max J. Volcansek, III, Ph.D.

100&
HEALTHY

Living Longer with
Phytomedicines from the
Republic of Georgia

W. SHAFFER FOX

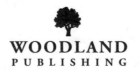

WOODLAND
PUBLISHING

Grateful acknowledgment is made to the following for use of these images: p.
27, Mark Page Fox; p. 30, Shaffer Fox and Louis Iglesias; p. 31, Nugzar
Kekelidze, Ph.D.; p. 32, Zakir Ramazanov, Ph.D.; p. 33, Gika Chelidze; p. 71,
Hungarian Patent Office; p. 72, Nugzar Kekelidze, Ph.D.; p. 124, Anna Britaeva
and Valentina Kolesnikova; p. 150, Capatah; p. 180, Nugzar Kekelidze, Ph.D.; p.
184 (left), Yuri Dobryakov, Ph.D.; p. 184 (center), Yuri Dobryakov, Ph.D.; p.
184 (right), Yuri Dobryakov, Ph.D.

Library of Congress Cataloging-in-Publication Data
Fox, W. Shaffer.
100 & healthy: living longer with phytomedicines from the Republic of
Georgia/ W. Shaffer Fox.
p.   cm.
Includes bibliographical references and index.
ISBN 1-58054-388-X (pbk.)
1. Longevity–Georgia (Republic) 2. Diet–Georgia (Republic) 3. Medicinal
plants–Georgia (Republic) 4. Roseroot–Georgia (Republic) 5.
Pomegranate–Georgia (Republic) 6. Blueberries–Georgia (Republic) 7.
Rhododendrons–Georgia (Republic) I. Title: One hundred and healthy. II. Title.
RA776.75.F69 2004
612.6'8'094758--dc22   2004016890

For ordering information, contact:
Woodland Publishing, 448 East 800 North, Orem, Utah 84097
(800) 777-2665
www.woodlandpublishing.com

Note: The information in this book is for educational purposes only and is not
recommended as a means of diagnosing or treating an illness. All matters concern-
ing physical and mental health should be supervised by a health practitioner
knowledgeable in treating that particular condition. Neither the publisher nor
author directly or indirectly dispenses medical advice, nor do they prescribe any
remedies or assume any responsibility for those who choose to treat themselves.

ISBN 1-58054-388-X

Printed in the United States of America

Contents

Preface

The republic of Georgia is one of the earth's most beautiful, bountiful, and historically significant nations. It is also one of the least understood. Yet, despite Georgia's relative obscurity in the minds of the American public, some North Americans who are interested in health and nutrition are becoming more aware of the country. They have heard that traditional Georgian people lived incredibly long lives.

Georgia is, in fact, renowned for having produced exceptionally high numbers of healthy centenarians—people who lived to be at least 100 years old. Perhaps no other country in the world has ever produced so many people who lived so long and in such good health. This so-called "Georgian longevity paradox" has attracted researchers for decades.

What caused this Georgian longevity? Scientists now believe they have found the answer, and it lies in the traditional Georgian diet.

Four potent plant species—most of them unique to

Georgia—have been regularly consumed by the longest-living Georgians for many centuries. These plants are *Rhododendron caucasicum*, Caucasian blueberry leaves, the Georgian pomegranate, and *Rhodiola rosea*, a plant not native to Georgia, but one that often was included in the diet there. Georgian and Russian scientists, among others, now believe that the frequent consumption of these plants was a primary cause of the extended health and longevity of traditional Georgians.

The four plants described in this book all contain natural chemicals that bring specific health benefits and fight aging. For example, all have been shown to protect DNA and slow the onset and progression of cancers and atherosclerosis, hardening of the arteries with plaque buildup on the interior arterial walls. More specifically, *Rhododendron caucasicum* is most often used to prevent and treat heart disease, arthritis and gout; it also helps prevent glaucoma. Caucasian blueberry leaves, the world's greatest source of specific chemicals that balance blood glucose levels, also reduce cholesterol and triglyceride levels and limit the damage caused by nitrites. The Georgian pomegranate is the best source of a chemical that prevents cancer cells from forming, kills those in existence, and inhibits cancer's spread. And *Rhodiola rosea* is most highly regarded for its effectiveness in preventing and treating depression and stress disorders, as well as improving mental and physical performance.

For thousands of years, each of these plants has been consumed by humans as part of their normal diets. For several hundreds of years, each has been successfully used in folk medicine. The plants have been subjects of intensive pharmacological and clinical research, and extracts of three of the four plants have been available over-the-counter and by prescription for more than fifty years. Hundreds of fortunate Westerners have learned of these plant extracts in recent years, and have used them with dramatic results. And yet because of past political turmoil and previously inadequate means of communication, these unique and important substances, which can help millions of people in the West, are still virtually unknown to Americans.

Now, after the fall of the Iron Curtain and with vast improvements in global communication, the intrinsic healthfulness of the traditional Georgian diet and lifestyle, and the foresight and brilliance of Georgian science, can be fully shared with the world. This book does that, outlining the traditional Georgian diet and providing countless studies that give evidence of each plant's health benefits.

Read these studies and try the plant extracts for yourself, as I have. You will find that they bring remarkable improvements, and you will come to understand the wisdom in traditional Georgian dietary practices. Ultimately, you will reap for yourself a happier, healthier, and longer life.

Acknowledgments

In presenting this book, I give special thanks to Zakir Ramazanov, Ph.D., who first introduced me to Georgia's great dietary traditions and the unique pharmacological activities of Caucasian phytomedicines.

I also wish to thank Nathela Chatara, executive director of the Georgian Association in Springfield, Ill. When all known potential sources of certain cultural materials had been exhausted, this perfect example of inherent Georgian friendliness and professionalism gladly put me in touch with select authorities within a single day.

Thanks to Merab Pachulia, M.S., a director of Georgian Opinion Research International in Tblisi, Georgia. He is a true gentleman and now a good friend, who acquired and provided an abundance of requested societal research reports, government data, permissions, and verifications. I would not have been able to obtain this information any other way. In addition, on at least fifteen occasions during the last few months of writing this book, Merab was the go-to guy who always came through. His intelligence, professionalism, contacts, and "get-it-done" mode of operation will always be appreciated. Merab loves Georgia, and he is another perfect example of what is so right and good about the country and its people.

Thank you Nick Erkomaishvili, operations manager of Caucasus Travel Ltd. in Tblisi, Georgia. During the final verification process for the book, Nick repeatedly made key contacts for me and provided translations that helped ensure the accuracy of the book. And thank you Professor Ether Kemertelidze, D.Sc, and Mr. Karen Mulkijanyan for your consistently enlightening correspondences and translations.

In addition, thanks go to: Gabriel D. Labbate, Ph.D., of Tblisi, Georgia, who rapidly provided difficult-to-find agricultural, linguistic, and census reports; American professor Jim Elliot, Ph.D.; Georgian/American professor Shota Vashakidze, Ph.D.; Georgian professors David Lordkipanidze, Ph.D., Ether Kemertelidze, D.Sc., and Nugzar Kekelidze, Ph.D.; Hungarian/Canadian professor Istvan Berczi, D.V.M., Ph.D.; Miklos Bendzsel, Ph.D., Eve Bakos, and Anna Balint of the Hungarian Patent Office; Lev Rubanov, Ph.D., and Yuri I. Dobryakov, Ph.D., of the Russian Academy of Sciences; Malgorzata Myc, M.S., of the University of Michigan; award-winning photographers Alexander Saakov, Gika Chelidze, M.A., and Gouram Tsibakhashvili; Lela Khartishvili of Caucasus Travel Ltd.; the reference department of the State Public Scientific Technical Library of the Siberian branch of the Russian Academy of Sciences; and Elena Zimina, Anna Britaeva, Olga Lavrik, Valentina Kolesnikova, Mark Page and Kelly Fox, Rocky Heinrich, and (again) Zakir Ramazanov, Ph.D., Merab Pachulia and Nick Erkomaishvili, each of whom obtained and provided one or more difficult-to-find photographs for this book.

I thank the several scientists and others who kindly gave their time to provide imperative verifications of data. In some cases, their contributions are cited in the text.

Thank you, Roy B. Kupsinel, M.D., Marjorie Smith, M.D., Rafael Avila, and Megan Vandre. During the writing of this book, they made important observations and recommendations for which I am very appreciative.

My appreciation to award-winning graphic artist Louis Iglesias, who consulted on many systems challenges and photography transfers.

Thank you Bob Howard, for forcing me to drop what I was doing and investigate what is proving to be the most beneficial source of phytonutrition on earth.

Thanks very much to Patricia Ann and Wilfred R. Fox, Louis and Bertha Shaffer, Nellie Cassidy, and Beth Snodgrass Amonette, who always have been there, and to my wonderful family— brother and sisters, in-laws, nieces and nephews, and friends old and new. Special thanks go out to Mary and Hank Mosher, Mark and Patrice Dillow, and Gorman, Freeman, Fox, Davis, Iglesias, Dabiere, Garrison, Gauthier, Staigers, Weber, Haber, Smith, Boyd, Frazier, Ed Dodge, Hughes, Jacobs, K. D., and Dr. Stewart White.

I am also grateful to the many renowned scientists who are increasingly performing valuable research on the substances presented here.

"May you have the good health and long life of a Georgian."

– Traditional Russian toast

Introduction

I first learned about *Rhododendron caucasicum* from a fax. A colleague, Bob Howard, sent it to me one day in 1997, but the original source of the one-page document was a nutritional products manufacturer in New York. The letter appeared to have been written by a foreigner.

Rhododendron caucasicum, it stated, was a plant indigenous to the republic of Georgia, a country famous for producing large numbers of centenarians. Georgians had used the substance for more than 2,000 years. Further, the plant supported all systems of the human body, and its efficacies had been demonstrated in clinical studies performed in both Russia and Georgia. Traditional Georgians considered *Rhododendron caucasicum*, called the Georgian snow rose, to be key to living a long and healthy life, the letter concluded.

A short time later Bob telephoned, very excited. "No one in the West seems to know about this *Rhododendron caucasicum*," he said. "It was a secret of the former Soviet Union. If this is a true key to healthy longevity, it could be one of the biggest stories in nutrition." Then Bob suggested I temporarily stop developing another nutritional product and begin investigating *Rhododendron caucasicum* full time.

I was instantly skeptical. "How were we lucky enough to have found out about this when no one else has?" I asked Bob somewhat sarcastically. Another colleague of ours had pried the story out of the New York manufacturer and sent it over, he said. Despite this explanation and Bob's enthusiasm, I wasn't interested. I was even a bit perturbed by his suggestion that I switch focus.

Over the next few days, Bob artfully riled on about Georgian longevity, antiaging, and *Rhododendron caucasicum* until logic demanded that I do some investigating. I decided to research the plant. Before I outline my research initiatives, though, I should explain the background within which I decided to move forward.

The World of Phytochemicals

During that time in 1997, excitement about the protective and healing effects of antioxidants was reaching storm level. In addition, new research revealing that phytochemicals— chemicals from plants—could fight cancer and protect the heart dominated the news. Each new study showed that the phytochemicals' protective and healing effects came primarily from their antioxidant activities.

This sudden barrage of health news about the benefits of phytochemicals provided information that was basic and nebulous at best. A report would come out one day proclaiming the cancer-inhibiting properties of an unnamed chemical in a certain fruit. The next day an almost unpronounceable chemical from a vegetable would be named, and doctors would say it "might prevent heart disease." This lack of detail created as much confusion across America as it did excitement. People didn't know what to believe, where to get more information, or how to find products that contained the correct phytochemicals. They also wondered why plants would produce these seemingly new chemicals. "What could plants possibly have in common with humans?" they asked.

One answer to that question is that plants need to protect their health, too. Plants are in constant danger. They are barraged by bacteria, viruses, fungi, ultraviolet radiation, oxidation (events that cause molecules to lose electrons), toxins, insects, worms, animals, humans, and extremes of cold, heat, moisture, and sunlight. And because plants are sedentary, they are more susceptible to these dangers than any other life forms. Therefore, over hundreds of millions of years, plants have developed the ability to produce unique, powerful, and protective chemicals to defend themselves.[1,2,3,4] These chemicals also give plants their color, flavor, smell, and texture.[1,4,5]

While many phytochemicals are not beneficial to humans,[5] scientists have identified thousands of protective chemicals, found in the 150,000-plus species of fruits and vegetables, which are beneficial.[5,6] These plant chemicals have become the basis for most modern medicines. In fact, in 2001 researchers at University of Iowa Health Care estimated that 75 percent of the world's medicines come from plants.[7]

Among the beneficial phytochemicals, there are many classes and subclasses. Probably the most exciting and well-known class is the phenolics. This class includes flavonoids, flavonals, catechins, isoflavones, and phenolic acids among its subclasses. In the flavonoid subclass alone, more than 5,000 phytochemicals have been discovered so far, and each one is an antioxidant that strengthens the human immune system, heals and protects the cardiovascular system, and slows the human aging process.[1,5]

When it comes to chemical composition, each species, subspecies, and variety of plant is unique. Furthermore, each part of a plant—flower, fruit, leaf, stem, or root—has its own unique chemistry as well. The chemical composition of each plant part varies with the seasons and with the plant's location. It also changes according to the stresses the plant must endure. These changes happen during a plant's life cycle as the chemicals within the plant react synergistically with each other to reduce certain chemicals or to produce even more protective chemicals in varying volumes.[2,4,5] The result is that during the springtime the leaves of a specific plant may contain high volumes of chemicals A and B, which are beneficial to humans, and low volumes of nonbeneficial chemicals D and E, which are not beneficial to humans. By the beginning of summer, however, the chemical makeup of the leaves may have changed so much that good chemicals A and B are almost nonexistent, and nonbeneficial chemicals D and E are present in high volumes.

The goal of nearly every plant biochemist and nutritionist is to discover a leaf, root, fruit, or other plant part with low volumes of nonbeneficial phytochemicals and very high volumes of beneficial phytochemicals—chemicals scientifically demonstrated to prevent and treat illnesses in humans. Once such a unique plant part is discovered, the challenge is to extract its phytochemicals in a manner that provides the highest possible amounts of the most important phytochemical(s). The final extract is processed further, bottled, and put on the market to improve the health of millions.

Finding such a plant part, let alone extracting it properly and successfully presenting it to the public, takes a great deal of time and research. But every few years or so, the ultimate dream of any plant biochemist or nutritionist comes true. With this hope in the back of my mind, I began investigating *Rhododendron caucasicum*.

The Path of Research

As I began my research, I hoped that *Rhododendron caucasicum*'s beneficial properties came from the antioxidant activities of phenolics. Like most scientists and at least some of the public, I was already familiar with phenolics' health benefits, so should this turn out to be true, it would simplify everything. However, initial library and Internet searches turned up nothing. So I had no choice but to go back to the original source of the information on *Rhododendron caucasicum*—the New York manufacturer.

I telephoned the manufacturing company, and a contact there told me that *Rhododendron caucasicum* was indeed a standardized phenolic extract. That thrilled me. He also confirmed that *Rhododendron caucasicum* extract was new to the United States, but because all research on the substance was written in Russian or Georgian, it may be weeks or months before translations could be completed. Nonetheless, he said, "One of the most credentialed scientists in the world—a man who is a Georgian, a former Soviet researcher, and a professor in the West—has validated the research." As it turned out, the fax Bob Howard sent me had actually been written by this scientist at the request of an international nutrients brokerage house.

Despite my requests, the manufacturer refused to name the scientist or the brokerage house backing this substance. Company leaders feared they could be cut out of future transactions if they did. However, I remained confident about

Rhododendron caucasicum's prospects, thanks to the simple fact that I knew this company was obsessed with documentation and analysis and had most likely investigated the plant thoroughly.

As an alternative to speaking with the foreign scientist, I requested that the company send me a sample of *Rhododendron caucasicum* extract, a certificate of analysis, and its research data—even if it were transcribed. I also submitted a series of questions about the plant. The first question pertained to the volume and types of phenolics in *Rhododendron caucasicum* extract. The second question was, "Is *Rhododendron caucasicum* wild crafted?" In other words, is it grown in the wild without the use of herbicides or pesticides? I asked this question because it had never made sense to me that nutritional products containing herbicides and pesticides, which cause diseases, be sold to people who wanted to prevent diseases. Besides, the use of herbicides and pesticides in farming has been shown to reduce the amount of phenolics in certain fruits by as much as 58 percent.[12]

My final question concerned extraction. I wanted to know whether the extraction process used with *Rhododendron caucasicum* involved toxic organic solvents. Such solvents, including acetone, chloroform, ethylacetate, and butanol, are commonly used in herbal extractions. They create powerful free radicals—unstable molecules that are missing some electrons and that damage other molecules because of it—in end products, and free radicals cause aging, cancer, and cardiovascular disease, among other detriments. Further, even if the amount of organic solvent residue in end products is in the parts per million or parts per billion, the accumulated buildup of these toxins in the body is damaging.

I hoped *Rhododendron caucasicum*'s beneficial chemicals were extracted without the use of toxic solvents, but I didn't expect that to be the case. In fact, to me that criterion seemed like an unattainable ideal. This was because, despite years of searching, I had never found a standardized herbal extract in the United States that had not utilized toxic solvents.

The next day the sample of *Rhododendron caucasicum* extract arrived from New York, along with a certificate of analysis. I was impressed. Whereas the total amount of phenolics was specified to be 40 percent, it tested at 49 percent; and whereas the total amount of taxifolins was specified to be 5 percent, high performance liquid chromatography (HPLC) method analysis showed it to be 5.9 percent. At that time, research already was confirming that taxifolins, a flavonoid, was proving to be amongst the most beneficial of all phenolics. Furthermore, the sample of *Rhododendron caucasicum* extract was devoid of pesticides and herbicides, and the substance had been extracted using a Russian-patented water and high pressure filtration technique—a technique that did not employ toxic solvents. Obviously, whoever directed the growth, harvesting, and extraction of *Rhododendron caucasicum* extract practiced perfection. He, she, or they were functioning far above the norms. That fact made me want to learn more.

Additional Testing

Thus far, the *Rhododendron caucasicum* extract sample had been evaluated using conventional testing methods. Scientists and manufacturers determine the integrity of nutritional substances and products through a variety of conventional testing methods, including: microbiological assaying, culture testing, HPLC method testing, atomic absorption spectrometry, nuclear magnetic resonance spectrometry, and other conventional state-of-the-art procedures. Conventional testing is essential and, for our safety, never should be neglected. An increasing number of companies, consumers, patients and health care practitioners, though, also rely on the natural testing arts of kinesiology and radionics, and I knew top experts in those fields.

I placed a few grams of *Rhododendron caucasicum* extract in a plastic bag and sent them to T.R. Edwards, a kinesiologist in Colorado. Three days later, T.R. called to report his results. "What is this *Rhododendron caucasicum?*" he exclaimed. "It's very strong. I've tested it on several people, and it seems to benefit every one of them."

Then I sent another sample of *Rhododendron caucasicum* to Jeff Levin, a top radionics authority in Ontario, Canada. Hundreds of Jeff's students, including several prominent M.D.'s and Ph.D.'s, successfully utilize his methods throughout the world. A few days later, Jeff called with his findings. "I get very strong readings from it," he said. "It's an amazing substance—very beneficial. On a scale of one to ten, with ten being the highest, it's a solid ten."

"It's rare to find something that tests this high," Jeff continued. "Can we get more of it?"

I immediately called Bob Howard and told him his intuitions about *Rhododendron caucasicum* were proving correct. If we could somehow contact the Georgian scientist who had developed the extract and convince him to quickly translate his clinical studies on *Rhododendron caucasicum*—and if the results of the clinical studies were as good as implied—we could have a longevity substance that would excel in every form of testing. And it would be a substance with a 2,000-year history.

But first we had to gain access to the Georgian scientist.

Dr. Zakir Ramazanov

In order to persuade the New York manufacturing company to give us the scientist's name, I had to prove that they would not be excluded from future transactions involving *Rhododenron caucasicum*. So I made the necessary legal arrangements that formed a limited alliance between the New York company and the Texas parent firm I was representing. Before the ink on the deal could dry, our contact at the manufacturing firm called from New York. "The name of the scientist you want to talk to is Dr. Zakir Ramazanov," he said.

Dr. Ramazanov's background was impressive. A native of Georgia, he not only spoke fluent English, but also communicated in Georgian, German, Russian, Spanish, Swahili, and Swedish. His academic credentials were outstanding. He was a top graduate of North Caucasian State University, with a double major in biochemistry and plant physiology. He shared the distinction of top graduate of the Soviet Academy of Sciences upon receiving his Ph.D. in plant physiology, and he was a two-time academic gold medalist. In addition, Ramazanov had been a senior scientist involved in space biology research at the Soviet Academy of Sciences. Then he went on to become chief of the Department of Biotechnology at the academy. He had worked as a professor at four Western universities, including Sweden's University of Umea, Spain's University of Las Palmas and University of Cordoba, and in the famous algae research labs of Louisiana State University. And he had published at least 140 research studies. On top of all that, he was also the man who introduced new methods for extracting beta carotene, letein, and lycopene.

But let me further impress upon you the significance of Dr. Ramazanov's credentials. In the former Soviet Union, less than one in five students was accepted to any of the nation's 900 colleges and universities.[9] Only a tiny fraction of those students were eventually accepted for graduate study at any of the nation's scientific academies and institutes. And only the absolute crème de la crème of graduate students could ever earn entry to the esteemed Soviet Academy of Sciences in Moscow, which was founded as the Academy of Arts and Sciences by Peter the Great in 1724 and which went on to become the single most important scientific institution in Russian and Soviet history. Because of this academy, Moscow is believed to have a greater concentration of mathematical talent than any other city in the world, and the academy's contributions to astronomy, rocketry, chemistry, physics, biomedical sciences, and biology are monumental and legendary.[9,10,11,12] Thus, Dr. Ramazanov's accomplishments—being a top graduate of the academy and head of its biotechnology department, not to mention his other advances—were truly amazing feats.

The strength of any science is only as good as its composer. Certainly, based upon what we already knew about Dr. Ramazanov and his longevity-promoting substance, *Rhododendron caucasicum*, we were about to embark on a top-notch project with one of the world's best.

I called Dr. Ramazanov a few days later and found him to be every bit as knowledgeable and accommodating as I had hoped. "I am always happy to talk about *Rhododendron caucasicum*," he said. "It's a symbol of my country. It's a symbol of my people." He assured me that the plant would help many Americans, then asked what I wanted to know. And thus began a relationship that has spanned more than seven years.

Starting from Georgian Roots

Over these past few years, I have spent countless hours on

the phone, transcribing Dr. Ramazanov's oral translations of clinical and pharmacological studies, repeatedly questioning and editing syntax, and reconfirming dates, study locations, participants, dosages, and results. During each conversation with Dr. Ramazanov and my own other research, my inner excitement has increased. It has long been apparent to me that *Rhododendron caucasicum* extract is, indeed, something very special. It is obviously a substance that can benefit millions of Americans and others by enhancing their chances at living long, healthy lives.

In addition, my association with Dr. Ramazanov and investigation of *Rhododendron caucasicum* has led me to learn of other extremely beneficial Georgian plants. These include Caucasian blueberry leaves, the Georgian pomegranate, and *Rhodiola rosea*, a plant not indigenous to Georgia, but from which many Georgian longevous have greatly benefited. Like

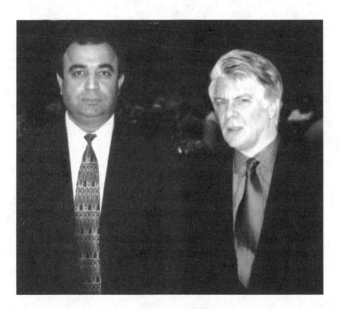

Zakir Ramazanov, Ph.D. (*left*), and the author

Rhododendron caucasicum, these plants are special chemical compositions that can improve the health of millions and lead to longer lives for all.

I have also come to realize that each of these plants is inextricably connected with Georgian history, culture, health, and longevity. They could not be fully appreciated without sufficient knowledge of the Georgian lifestyle. That's why I now believe that the best way to learn about *Rhododendron caucasicum* and the other three plants also used by traditional Georgians is to begin by investigating everything Georgian—including Georgian longevity. That's the route I pursued, and it has led me to confirm my belief in these plants' benefits.

CHAPTER 1

Georgia and Georgian Longevity

The republic of Georgia is an ancient land with an astonishing history and intrinsically healthful customs. But for nearly a thousand years, its true magnificence has been mostly obscured from the world by differences in language, worship, and politics. In fact, today few Americans know much of anything about the country, and they often confuse it with the state of Georgia. Therefore, a fundamental knowledge of Georgia is necessary before the traditional Georgian lifestyle and diet can be fully appreciated.

Prior to 1997, almost all I knew about Georgia was that it was located in the heart of the Caucasus Mountain region. I knew its people had an ancient and glorious history entwined with the Greeks, Romans, and other classical civilizations, but also that the Georgians had a unique lifestyle and wore unique clothes. I knew Georgians were predominantly Orthodox Christian, whereas most of their bordering neighbors practiced Islam. And finally, I knew the Georgians, along

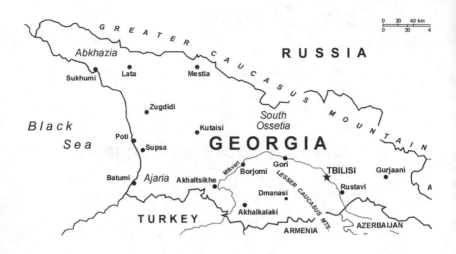

Map of the republic of Georgia

with some of their non-Russian neighbors in the Caucasus, ate a lot of yogurt and purportedly lived very long lives.

When I began investigating Georgia in earnest, I found out much more. I learned about its topography, cultural traditions, resources, economic structure, and history. Most important, I gained factual knowledge about the intricacies of the Georgian diet, Georgian medicinal practices, and the phenomenon of Georgian longevity. What follows is thus an overview of what I have come to know about this amazing country and its people.

An Introduction to Georgia

Georgia is located about 5,400 miles east of Boston. Positioned between the Black and Caspian seas, it is separated from southern Russia by the Caucasus Mountains. The country's balmy, palm-dotted beaches at times lay only miles from massive snowcapped mountains—mountains that pierce the clouds and are surrounded by high-altitude forests of extraordinary vegetation. Three of Georgia's mountains, Shkhara, Janqi, and Kazbek, soar more than 2,000 feet higher than the tallest mountains in the U.S.'s forty-eight contiguous states.[1]

Georgia's borders contain an astonishing twenty-three soil-climatic zones, and consequently, in their diversity and composition, the country's unique plant species significantly differ from the plants in bordering neighbor countries. Today, 4,200 species of vascular plants grow in Georgia, and the country is home to thousands more species of lesser vegetation. Most amazing is that of the vascular plants, 380 (9 percent) are native to Georgia, and 600 (14.2 percent) are native to the Caucasus region in which Georgia is located.[2]

Visitors to Georgia amply attest to the nation's spectacular and unparalleled beauty. Its unique architecture, cultural

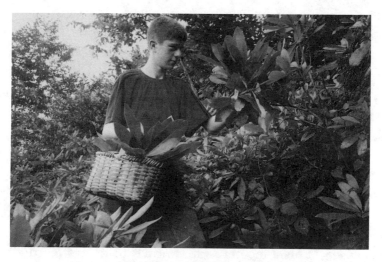

A young Georgian collecting large mature
Rhododendron caucasicum leaves

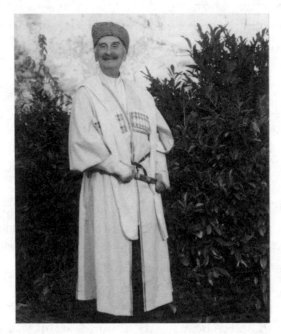

A Georgian in traditional dress in front of Caucasian blueberry plants

attractions, and topography spellbind everyone, regardless of past travel and living experiences. The tourists are amazed, for example, by the distinctive, alluring, and mystical qualities of traditional Georgian music and dance. These arts, along with the country's native garments, have survived centuries. Also, they learn that traditional Georgian cuisine is considered to be the most delicious and healthful on earth. And they find that the nation's rich history comes alive in the country's 12,000 monuments and museums.[3]

Georgia's greatest attraction, of course, is its people. Georgian tradition says guests are sent from God, and because of this, Georgians are known to be among the most hospitable people on earth. In addition, visitors find the Georgian people to be exceptionally intelligent, hard work-

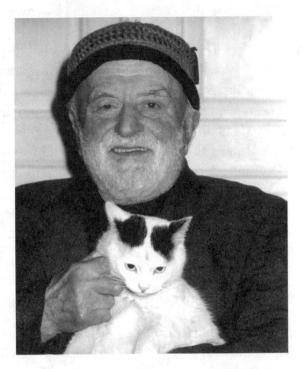

102-year-old Georgian Pavel Abuladze and friend

ing, friendly, and chivalrous, and the society highly educated and motivated.[3,4,5]

The hundreds of tribes inhabiting Georgia in 79 A.D. spoke just as many different languages,[6] but today, there is one official Georgian language. It is taught in Georgian schools and used in commerce, and it is well over 2,000 years old. The Georgian alphabet, created during the third century B.C., is one of only fourteen alphabets of the world, despite the fact that Georgians make up only about 1/1,700 of humanity and the nation is less than half the size of Iowa.[3,7] Some believe the language's crescent-shaped symbols could have emerged from Aramaic, the Semitic dialect Jesus spoke.[8] Today,

Assyrian Neo-Aramaic is still spoken by about 3,000 Georgians.[9]

Georgia also has a wealth of natural resources. It possesses numerous warm water ports and advanced transportation and communication systems. And it has nearly completed its conversion to the free market system. Thanks to these and other factors, Georgia's economy is becoming strong. In fact, economically, Georgia is the fastest growing of all former Soviet republics. Continued, dramatic economic growth is projected for the country's future.[3,10] Thus, probably no nation with as troubled a political past as Georgia's is more prepared to flourish, and thereby benefit all humankind, during the years to come.

GEORGIA'S EARLIEST ROOTS

In recent years, scientists and others have concluded that Georgia was the site of one of the earth's earliest civilizations. This conclusion comes through a mention of Georgia in one of Western civilization's creation myths and through archaeological findings.

The mythological connection appears in Greece. Ancient Greece's early creation myth includes Zeus' punishment of Prometheus on Mount Caucasus in Georgia. Of this connection, Robert D. Kaplan wrote in *The Atlantic Monthly,* "The very antiquity of the Prometheus story . . . could be further evidence that the Caucasus was a cradle of civilization."[8] Kaplan went on to point out that even the Western name for the land, "Georgia," probably comes from the Greek word "geo," which means "earth," and that on their first visits to Georgia, ancient Greeks were amazed to see many people working the land.[8]

From archaeologists' point of view, one of the first finds

that led to this conclusion came during the 1980s, when the most primitive of stone tools were found beneath a tiny medieval castle in Dmanisi, Georgia.[10] An early human jaw-bone was discovered at the same site in 1991, and an early human foot bone was unearthed there in 1997. However, when these bones were dated, the scientific community disputed the results: The bones were just too old to have been found outside Africa, the site of the world's oldest unearthed early human remains.

A 1999 discovery at the same site put an end to the skepticism. That summer, a team of scientists from Germany and Georgia unearthed a complete early human cranium and a skullcap from a second early human.[11] The cranium and skullcap were subsequently dated to 1.7 million years of age,[12,13] and at the time, Carl C. Swisher III, Ph.D., then of the Berkeley Geochronology Center, told the Associated Press that the dating had been confirmed by three different methods.[14] This dating meant that the partial skulls, which scientists believed came from an early human species between *Homo ergaster* and *Homo erectus,* were the oldest human ancestral fossils of their species ever found outside Africa.[14,15]

In late 2001, another early human skull and jaw bone were found at the Dmanisi site, and the discoveries were reported in *Science* magazine[16] and *National Geographic* (in a ten-page cover story).[17] This third skull and jaw bone dated to at least 1.7 million years of age as well and appeared to come from an even earlier species of humans than the others. Significantly, no other site outside Africa has provided such a large collection of ancient human remains even half this age.[18]

Additional archaeological evidence shows how early humans flourished in Georgia. Humanoid-inhabited cave sites dating to between 100,000 B.C. and 40,000 B.C. can be found along the seashores, as well as in the inland and highland areas of Georgia.[19,20] Ongoing excavations indicate that substantial water supplies and lush vegetation have been abundant in Georgia for millions of years, and the cultivation of fruits and vegetables in Georgia can be traced back to between 7,000 B.C. and 5,000 B.C.[2,21,22] This proof of agricultural know-how and evidences of the early domestication of animals are hallmarks of civilization in Georgia that predate Greek[23,24] and perhaps even Mesopotamian cultures.[8] Research also reveals that between 5,000 B.C. and 4,000 B.C. Georgians began using metal tools.[21,25] By 3,000 B.C. they had learned to alloy copper and tin into bronze,[23] and by 1,500 B.C. Georgian metallurgy and pottery were flourishing and renowned.[19,26]

GEORGIA'S MEDICINAL HISTORY

In addition to being a cradle of civilization, Georgia has also long been recognized for its people's skill in medicine and healing. This connection comes through Greek mythology and other historical sources.

From Greek myths, we learn that Jason and the Argonauts went to Georgia to retrieve the Golden Fleece. Once they arrived there, Medea, the daughter of the Colchis king Aeëtes of Georgia, fell in love with Jason, helped retrieve the Golden Fleece, and fled with Jason back to Greece. Many of the Argonauts were injured during the escape, and Medea skillfully treated them with Georgian herbal medicines. Thus, Georgian folk etymologists believe the word "medicine" is derived from the name Medea—the name of one of "the first [believed] to use plants for their curative powers," according to Darra Goldstein, a professor of Russian at Williams College.[27] Medea's mother, Gekat, purportedly was an expert pharmacist as well.[28,29]

Historically, there are several other indications of Georgia's long-standing skill in medicine. Hippocrates (b. 460 B.C.), who is called the father of medicine, wrote how impressed he was with the healthful diet and customs he witnessed during a visit to Georgia. And the Roman poet Horace mentioned the unique medications Georgians used in his writings.[30] These references show that Georgia's medical tradition dates back hundreds and even thousands of years.

But there are some slightly more recent indications of Georgia's medical prowess as well. One comes in the *Karabadini*, Georgian medical books written during the Middle Ages.[23,29,30] These books include instructions based on centuries of Georgian medicinal practices. Even then—hundreds of years before vaccination was discovered in other parts of the world—Georgian folk doctors were vaccinating people for diseases such as smallpox. Another even more recent indication is a partial medical inventory published in the early 1800s that lists 569 medications known in Georgia. Three hundred seventy-two of these medications were prepared from plants.[29,31] Georgians regularly consumed many of these plants as part of their daily diets, and in many cases, they simply consumed more of these plants during times of illness.[32] The result of all this medical know-how has been a preponderance of healthy centenarians in Georgia.

Thus, throughout history, Georgians have been known for their unique lifestyle, diet, and advanced knowledge of plants and plant medicines. They have a centuries-old reputation for good health and longevity.

Georgian Longevity

What are the reasons for the Georgian longevity phenomenona? Are these plants alone responsible for Georgian longevity, or are other factors involved? And does the healthy longevity of pre-modern Georgians still exist today? To find the answers to these questions, I consulted Sula Benet's groundbreaking book *How to Live to Be 100: The Lifestyle of the People of the Caucasus,* the 1973 *National Geographic* article "Every Day Is a Gift When You Are Over 100," and several detailed research reports.

Reviewing these prior investigations quickly yielded interesting considerations and revelations. Most notably, and to my surprise, the tremendous Georgian longevity of centuries past has become a victim of the modern age and is on the decline—a problem I'll discuss shortly. But also, although there is substantial evidence that the longevity of "traditional" Georgians—those who have adhered to older customs and practices—was caused by these people's lifestyle and diet, many theorists still profess that it was the result of other factors, perhaps multiple factors working in concert. Some of the factors they cite are genetics, Georgian intelligence, and the altitude at which Georgians live. When these factors are examined in detail, however, it is clear that none can fully account for Georgian longevity.

POTENTIAL FACTORS IN GEORGIAN LONGEVITY

Genetics. Some theorists propose that Georgian longevity comes through the propagation of a good health/longevity gene. However, if this were the case, all inheritors of such an unusual gene would have connected ancestries—an unlikely possibility already eliminated by genetic research.[33]

A review of Georgia's diverse history also refutes the genetic theory. For well over a million years, Georgia has been traversed by various groups of humans and their early human predecessors.[12] Since about 2,000 B.C. or 3,000 B.C., Georgian bloodlines have mixed with the bloodlines of visitors from many lands, including Europe, Eurasia, and the Mediterranean.[34] And between the first and seventeenth centuries, Georgia was invaded by the Romans, the Persians, the Mongols, the Tartars, the Iranians, and the Turks (who invaded repeatedly). In addition, in 1801, Georgia, then a nearly surrounded Orthodox Christian outpost, sought protection from Orthodox Christian Russia and was annexed by Tsar Paul.[35] Of course, by then, Russian bloodlines had already been diluted by the conquering Cimmerians, Scythians, Sarmatians, Avars, Goths, Khazars, Bulgars, and Vikings.[36] Since that time, Georgia has been and continues to be a preferred dwelling place for people of many lands and bloodlines.[32,37] Modern Georgians reportedly now represent more than 80 different nationalities,[38] and today, seven major languages and more than 200 minor languages and dialects are spoken as "mother tongues" in Georgia.[39] Therefore, the genetic theory must be tempered by the fact that there has been as much mixing of genes in Georgia as nearly anywhere else on earth.[33]

Intelligence. Other theorists have speculated that longevity is linked to brain power—that having a brain that functions at optimum levels indicates and promotes healthy physiology. This theory is quite promising, given Georgia's educated population.

Georgians are generally very intelligent. This is evidenced by the fact that the country's population has been well educated for years, both before and during Georgia's time as part of the former Soviet Union. In the Soviet Union, education was mandatory and particularly rigorous. Instructors drove students to excel academically, not simply for student self-achievement and gratification, but also to meet the needs and expectations of the motherland.[40,41,42] As part of that Soviet system, Georgians therefore also excelled. In fact, of all the former Soviet republics, including Russia, Georgia produced the highest proportion of students who qualified for higher education and secured college degrees.[43] Each of these students was fluent in at least two languages, Georgian and Russian.[44]

But Georgia had a highly developed educational system and linguistic tradition long before it became a part of the Soviet Union.[40] As noted above, cultures, identities, and bloodlines have been extremely fluid in Georgia and the Caucasus since ancient times. Ronald G. Suny, Ph.D., Professor of Political Science at the University of Chicago, in a conference report for the Berkeley Program for Soviet and Post-Soviet Studies, wrote that Georgia has always been "a highly differentiated population living with [dozens of] mutually non-intelligible languages."[45] In another conference report for the same institution, Leanne Hinton, Ph.D., Professor of Linquistics at the University of California, Berkeley, wrote that the Caucasus is one of the rare places on earth where languages "have tended to accumulate over time rather than replace each other."[46] Therefore, as Suny goes on to point out, learning the languages of one's neighbors has been the norm—indeed, a necessity—in the Caucasus for thousands of years.[45] Today, Georgia's literacy rate is 99 percent,[47] and nearly all adult Georgians speak both Georgian and Russian, and an estimated 10 to 20 percent of all Georgians speak English, German, or French.[48] An estimated 50 percent of Georgian students speak English.[49]

New research shows that there is, in fact, a correlation between higher education/high linguistic ability in early life and slightly longer life spans, although some biological predisposition may be involved.[50-53] Despite these promising results, however, the intelligence factor cannot fully account for Georgian longevity. The longer life spans that seem related to intelligence simply aren't long enough to account for the several years of additional life that many traditional Georgians experienced.

Altitude. Another theory is that Georgian longevity is due to the high altitude at which much of the nation lives. More specifically, some postulate that humans who live at high altitudes exist on less oxygen and, therefore, suffer from less cell oxidation, or free-radical damage, than those living at lower altitudes. Cell oxidation is defined as any event during which a molecule gains too much oxygen, loses too much hydrogen, or is otherwise caused to lose electrons.

On the surface, this theory and others related to oxygen levels at high altitudes might seem to make sense. However, scientists have found little correlation between long life and high altitude environments. Besides that, there is no indication that residents of Butte, Montana, or Bogota, Columbia, for example, live appreciably longer lives than residents of Portsmouth, Virginia or Rio de Janeiro, Brazil. Thus, altitude alone cannot be the cause of Georgian longevity.

I suspect that some additional factors may be entwined with the altitude theory. The fact is, Georgians living at higher altitudes are more likely to be physically active and adhere to the traditional Georgian lifestyle and diet. These Georgians have exhibited the greatest health and longevity.[39,54]

LONGEVITY'S MOST PROBABLE CAUSE

While genetics, intelligence, and altitude may have contributed somewhat to the high percentage of Georgian centenarians, none of these factors, nor all three combined, could have produced traditional Georgians' tremendous longevity. After all, none of these characteristics is unique to Georgia. And yet, long-living Caucasians, most notably the Georgians, have been amply chronicled almost as oddities of nature by the Greeks, Iranians, Arabians, Russians, and others long before and many times since the 1917 October Revolution.[55] These people's longevity, then, must come from a unique source.

As will become apparent in the following chapters, and as I've learned during the last several years, the traditional Georgian dietary lifestyle is the one and only factor unique and powerful enough to have produced disproportionately high numbers of healthy Georgian centenarians. This matchless, healthful diet has been noted throughout the span of history, and now, I believe it provides such complete nutrition, such protection against precursors to illness, and such healing action that long, healthy living should be the natural result of its observance in any society.

But there is also another reason why the Georgian diet is the most probable cause of the country's unusual longevity. This reason is related to the second question I raised about longevity, namely, does the healthy longevity of pre-modern Georgians still exist today? The answer is no. In fact, the concentration of Georgian centenarians per capita has been declining for the last several decades. At the same time, while genetic trends and intelligence/linguistic ability remained near constant in the republic of Georgia, there have been several deleterious changes to Georgian lifestyle—including the replacement of much of the traditional Georgian diet with common Western-style foods and beverages. Thus, diet and lifestyle are the only factors that explain both the unusual longevity and its recent decline. The healthful diet protected against aging-related illnesses and thereby extended longevity, and deleterious changes in lifestyle and diet reduced longevity.

DECLINING GEORGIAN LONGEVITY: A CLOSER LOOK

As just mentioned, modern research indicates that the concentration of Georgian centenarians per capita has been declining. Some of the decline—possibly about 10 percent—can be attributed the previous century's many wars, wherein thousands of Georgians, who might otherwise be counted among the centenarians today, were lost. Since 1924,

Table 1. Longevity Trends in the Republic of Georgia

	Population	People over 100 years of age	Ratio
Rep. of Georgia 1926	2,677,200	4,301	1 in 622
Rep. of Georgia 1959	4,044,000	2,080	1 in 1,944
Rep. of Georgia 1970	4,728,205	1,849	1 in 2,564
Rep. of Georgia 1979	4,993,182	907	1 in 5,505
Rep. of Georgia 1989	5,400,841	1,048	1 in 5,153
Rep. of Georgia 2000	4,604,200	1,132	1 in 4,067
Rep. of Georgia 2002	4,409,800	658	1 in 6,701

Sources: DSG (Department of Statistics, Republic of Georgia). 2002.[61] Census Department of Georgia. 2002a,b.[62,63]

between 385,000 and 425,000 Georgians have perished as a result of wars and political unrest.[56-60] However, the balance of the decline—about 90 percent of it—results from other, reversible factors.

What are these factors? As noted, research strongly indicates a link between the unique Georgian diet and longevity. In addition, the Georgians themselves believe their ancestors' tremendous longevity was the result of lifestyle and diet. Therefore, we must look for deleterious changes in these areas as the primary mitigating factors to current Georgian longevity.

Farming trends. During Georgia's Soviet period, from 1921 through mid-1991, the Soviet Union collectivized thousands of small farms into massive plantations. The Soviets also replaced many important species of fruits and vegetables found only in Georgia with a few foreign species that produced higher yields per acre and/or that had more appetizing appearances.[2] In fact, to understand how completely Georgian species were replaced by Soviet-dictated ones, note that although Georgia comprised less than 1/322 of the former Soviet Union's land area and although nearly 80 percent of Georgia is covered by mountains and 40 percent by forests, Georgia produced 97 percent of the Soviet empire's citrus fruits, 93 percent of its tea, and imperative harvests of other fruits, vegetables, and grains, plus important outputs of dairy products.[9,64,65] Of the medicinal plants that survived this change to plantation farming, many were thenceforth lost as land was overharvested or cleared.[2] Today, only about 10 percent of the region's endemic vegetation remains.[66]

Eventually, over a period of several decades, knowledge of the characteristics of these medicinal plants was lost as well. However, some of the lost species of Georgian fruits and vegetables, including species of medicinal plants, have been saved in seed bank collections at research and extension centers. These species could therefore be replanted one day and again provide benefits.[2]

Fortunately, two of Georgia's three most important medicinal plants, which are presented in the following chapters, grow wild at high elevations. Because of this, they were not overharvested, nor were they replaced by other plant species. The third important plant discussed here, though not a high-altitude species, was not replaced either. Even so, the healing properties of these three plants, like the properties of many Georgian medicinal plants, have been forgotten by nearly all but a few scientists and lay people.[2] I noted this during a long discussion about *Rhododendron caucasicum* and alpine tea with a prominent middle-aged Georgian friend. After I described *Rhododendron caucasicum* and alpine tea for some time, he said, "Wait, now I think I know what you're talking about. Yes. My grandmother used to have me drink that tea when I would have a fever or the flu as a child. Yes, I remember. It worked very well. What happened to it?"[67]

Medical trends. As Georgian farms were being collectivized into high-output plantations, the Soviets also set up socialized/state-run medical facilities throughout the region. These new or converted hospitals, clinics, first-aid stations, and pharmacies practiced and dispensed modern Soviet-style medicine. They were directed from central planning offices in Moscow.[68] This change in the medical system meant that people increasingly began to rely on modern pharmacology to heal their ills instead of using traditional Georgian plant medicines—which were themselves disappearing. This further lessened the use and knowledge of Georgian folk medicine and of important Georgian medicinal plants.

On the positive side, the Soviets subsequently became very interested in Georgian folk medicines and indigenous plants. In fact, Soviet pharmaceutical and clinical studies have since provided a wealth of information about the effects of Georgian medicinal plants.[39,69] Additionally, the Georgian Academy of Science's Institute of Pharmacochemistry has been conducting expeditions to discover, collect, register, and study plant species currently growing in Georgia. The institute has developed several testing fields where various medicinal plants' growth requirements can be studied. From there the plants are made available to biologists, chemists, plant physiologists, pharmacologists and others for further analysis. Of about four hundred plants studied so far, ninety-five structurally new organic substances have been discovered, and dozens of medicines have been developed from them.[30] These outcomes are indications of Georgia's past and future potential in the medical world.

At the same time, however, it is also important to note that some of the surviving plants, as well as many of the lost plants, were part of the traditional Georgian diet. Now, unfortunately, in most cases, the surviving medicinal plants are consumed as medicines only *after* a person becomes ill.[39,69]

Food trends. The traditional Georgian diet primarily consisted of fresh, potent, nutrient-dense fruits and vegetables, many of which were unique to the Caucasus. It also included nutrient-rich yogurts and other milk products, lean meats, medicinal teas, phenolic-rich wines, and mineral-rich glacial water. Chemical preservatives were unheard of, and honey, not refined sugar, was used as a sweetener. In addition, traditional Georgians rarely canned or stored foods; leftovers were either immediately shared with neighbors or discarded.

In contrast, since the 1960s, sugary pastries, soft drinks, and foods containing preservatives have all worked their way into

Table 2. Food Products & Percent of Georgian Homes in
Which They're Found

Sunflower oil	79.7%	Macaroni	62.1%
Butter	51.9%	Margarine	41.9%
Chocolate	32.1%	Salami, sausage, etc.	31.7%
Mayonnaise	24.0%	Packaged flour	21.9%
Biscuits	16.8%	Canned fish	14.8%
Ready paste	10.2%		

Source: *Georgian Opinion Research Business International, 2000*[72]

Georgia. Increasingly, these foods are consumed by nearly all of the populace, including many of the elderly.[70]

Research shows that when sugar-laden or otherwise unhealthy foods are consumed, they typically replace beneficial foods that protect and support good health.[71] This is certainly true of Georgians. A survey of the populace conducted in 2000 showed that modern conveniences have, in fact, replaced much of the traditional Georgian diet, which was so supportive of good health and longevity.

Eighty-five percent of Georgians now drink non-medicinal teas every day, and these are usually sweetened with refined sugar. Sixty-one percent consume Turkish coffee every day, and 44 percent consume instant coffee daily. In addition, the consumption of yogurt is at an all-time low. And only 16 percent of Georgians still drink mineral water daily.[39,67,72]

Urban migration. A dramatic Georgian migration has taken place in recent years, with large numbers of people moving from the nation's rural areas—where the greatest concentrations of centenarians existed—to its cities. Between 1979 and

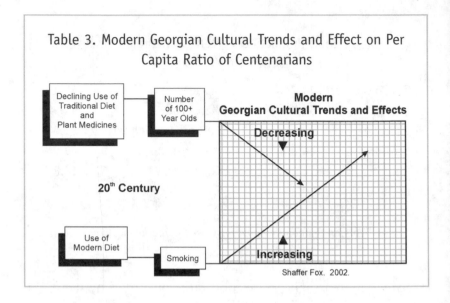

Table 3. Modern Georgian Cultural Trends and Effect on Per Capita Ratio of Centenarians

Shaffer Fox. 2002.

1989, Georgia's population grew 8.16 percent.[73,74,75] During the same time period, the country's urban populations grew 16.7 percent, while rural populations grew only 0.3 percent.[73]

Converting from rural life to city life almost requires that many cultural traditions, including healthy dietary practices, be abandoned, as access to natural, traditional ingredients is limited. This would surely affect the concentration of centenarians in Georgia. In addition, moving from idyllic, rural Georgia to the country's cities limits regular contact with life-long friends, induces stress, and makes one subject to the dangers of city life—all of which would also affect longevity.

Smoking. Cigarette smoking has become widespread in Georgia. Surveys show that more than 33 percent of the population currently smokes extremely strong cigarettes,[72] and the incidence of smoking in the country appears to be increasing. Of course, as is also now well known, cigarette smoking is the biggest preventable cause of illness and death in the modern world. It has claimed more than 100 million lives during the twentieth century alone.[77]

Setbacks in the health care system. Like most other former Soviet republics, Georgia faced severe problems after it gained its independence from the Soviet Union (in May 1991). One of these was a dramatic decline in the availability of state-of-the-art health care. In fact, government expenditures for health care during 1994 were less than 10 percent of those in 1990. Between 1991 and 1996, the overall general health of the population suffered tremendously: Infant mortality rose by 13 percent, and age-adjusted mortality rose by 18 percent.[43,75]

In July 1995, the Georgian government passed legislation to restructure the nation's health care system. The government allowed for and even promoted private ownership of most state-owned health service facilities, including pharmacies, clinics, and most hospitals. By January 31, 1998, 10,515 of the 10,656 government operations slated for privatization had been successfully privatized, and 541 of these businesses were providing health-related services. These are new businesses, though, in an ancient country but a new nation strapped for cash.[43,75] Consequently, medical analysis, interventions, and countermeasures—which are constantly improving in the West—have stagnated in Georgia.[76]

The deficit in conventional health care occurred when Georgians were already increasingly replacing their traditional diet with foods that provide little nutrition (and could even be harmful), when widespread smoking had already begun to debilitate the population, and when the cumulative effects of nearly total changes in lifestyle were becoming manifest.

Considering these difficulties, it's not surprising that modern longevity rates in Georgia have been declining for decades.

REVISITING LONGEVITY'S MOST PROBABLE CAUSE

In the final analysis, it is clear that only two factors can explain both Georgians' unique longevity and the recent decline in the country's numbers of centenarians. Those factors are the observance or neglect of the traditional Georgian diet and lifestyle.

In the West today, advancing medical analysis, interventions, and countermeasures are primarily responsible for extending people's longevity. But until recently in Georgia, longevity had always been supported by the unique, protective, traditional Georgian diet and the country's indigenous plant medicines, so supportive of good health. One easily can imagine the benefits that could come through combining modern medicine with the protective diet and medicines of pre-modern Georgians. That's why next I'll explore the Georgian diet in more detail—to begin to explain how to adapt this diet to modern lifestyles.

CHAPTER 2

The Georgian Diet

"Of all factors affecting functions of human physiology, diet is one of the most important," wrote Sula Benet in *How to Live to Be 100: The Lifestyle of the People of the Caucasus.*[1] Georgians have long believed this. Traditional Georgians, in particular, always believed that the quality of one's diet was a determining factor in the quality and length of one's life. From ancient times, they consumed specific foods to ensure proper nutrition, maintain good health, and prevent illnesses.

Georgian Ideas About Food

The basic Georgian diet included a diverse array of foods and remained unchanged for more than two thousand years, or until the early twentiethth century. Essentially, to eat as a traditional Georgian meant to eat only the freshest of good foods—clean foods full of color, flavor, and nutrients. These foods primarily included fresh vegetables and fruits—often of unique species—and also lean meats, dairy products and herbal and mineral beverages.[2]

Georgian centenarians' diet remained virtually unchanged through the years because the people valued consistency in what they ate. So, although foreign visitors to Georgia introduced many new foods, this fare was consumed only in moderation (until recently). Georgian centenarians considered new foods to be interesting and infrequent adjuncts to, rather than replacements for, their traditional diet. Their idea was that maintaining a consistent diet of the same fresh and nutrient-dense foods, eaten in moderation at about the same times every day, produced a natural rhythm in the body and thereby reduced stress on both body and mind. To maintain this rhythm, Georgians didn't allow themselves to become excessively hungry. In fact, in preparation for travel, they would eat before their departure, because healthy foods might not be available during the journey and because arriving at a destination hungry might make them more likely to overindulge.[2,3]

In addition to valuing consistency in their diets, traditional Georgians approached mealtimes in an interesting way. They thought of these occasions as relaxed, pleasurable breaks during busy days and nights, and as centerpieces for festive events. Basically, mealtimes were for regeneration. This came through nutritional replenishment and emotionally uplifting conversation. Reading, telling sad stories, or arguing while eating were considered bad table manners; these actions were depressing and unhealthy. In addition, eating quickly was frowned upon, so traditional Georgian meals were never rushed.[2,3]

As previously mentioned, Georgians believed that a good meal did not have to be a big meal. To Georgians, a person who overindulged on food or alcohol was boring, shameful, and emotionally confused. As Sula Benet wrote, "Georgians believed that a person should be able to 'eat at nine different tables' per day, but that they should eat only enough to satisfy their hunger."[3] Additionally, Georgians believed a person should be able to drink wine with every post-breakfast meal and during every gathering, but never become drunk.[4]

Interestingly, the results of several scientific studies from the last century seem to indicate that these Georgians probably also prolonged their lives by limiting their food intake. Research indicates that they would have been less prone to heart attacks, for one thing. After all, a 2000 study led by Harvard Medical School researcher Fransicso Lopez-Jimenez, M.D., showed that the risk of a heart attack increases by 400 percent during the hours immediately following consumption of a heavy meal.[5] In addition, traditional Georgians' propensity for eating nutrition-rich, low calorie meals seems to have affected their overall physiology as well, given other research results. For example, Dr. Clive McKay's experiments at Cornell University in the 1930s showed that reducing caloric intake early in life prolonged the rats' most active years of life.[6,7] And dozens of subsequent controlled studies on other species have produced similar results.[8,9] One of those studies, by Drs. Weindruch and Walford, was the first to show 10 percent to 20 percent increases in mean and maximum survival times with reduced caloric intake—even when subjects' calorie reduction didn't begin until middle age.[10] Additional studies on primates are currently underway at the University of Wisconsin, the University of Maryland, and the National Institute on Aging,[11] and although these studies won't be completed for several years, an early report from Wisconsin indicates that calorie reduction has already slowed the onset of some age-related physiologic changes.[12,13]

Along with moderate food consumption, lean physiques

and exercise were the norm in Georgia. Traditional Georgians said a person must be physically active throughout his or her early life and middle years in order to remain active later in life. And in general, Georgians considered lazy, overweight, or obese people to be ill.[2]

Finally, traditional Georgians thought diet could help control both the severity and duration of illnesses. As proof of this notion, Sula Benet cited a Georgian medical guide written in the eleventh century. It stated: "Most sicknesses are intensified by food. A small sickness can develop into a large one, depending on what the sick person eats. The doctor should prescribe the diet along with medication. The important thing is that a sick person should eat very light food."[14]

Constituents of the Georgian Diet

Now that Georgians' basic ideas about food have been set forth, the specifics of the Georgian diet can be explored. As mentioned above, the core of the traditional diet was eating fresh, good foods rich in color and nutrients. But in addition, some unique ingredients in the Georgian diet specifically encouraged good health and longevity. Four of these were specific plants with tremendous health benefits. They will be discussed in the remainder of the book. Some of the other beneficial elements of the diet are outlined below.

GEORGIAN WINE

Georgians have a legendary love for wine that is based on their ancient tradition of grape cultivation. In fact, scientists have determined that the original species of wine grape and the earliest known cultured grape varieties first grew in the

Caucasus region, where Georgia is located.[2,15,16,17] Archaeologists have unearthed wine presses and related utensils in Georgia that indicate that wine making has been practiced in the country for more than 4,000 years. In addition, they have found accumulations of grape seeds from cultivated vines that have been carbon dated to between 7,000 B.C. and 5,000 B.C.[16,17,18] But beyond the archaeological evidence of Georgia's wine-making tradition, there is also historical evidence. Some celebrities of antiquity, such as Apollo of Rhodes, Procopius of Caesaria, and Xenophon professed their love for Georgia's special nectar wines.[2,19,20] And sometime between the eighth and twelfth centuries B.C., Homer wrote in his epic poem *The Odyssey* of the "fragrant wine" in the land that is Georgia.[2,20] Additionally, linguists believe that the words *vin, vine, vino, Wein,* and *wine* are derivatives of the Georgian word *ghvino/gvino.*[17,20] Approximately five hundred varieties of grapes have been recorded in Georgian scientific literature, and today at least three hundred of those local varieties still exist in Georgia.[21,22]

One of the great things about wine is that it possesses free-radical-neutralizing phenolics—which, to reiterate from the Introduction, are beneficial plant chemicals that act as antioxidants to strengthen the immune system, heal and protect the cardiovascular system, and slow the aging process. However, as was also mentioned previously, the antioxidant activity of fruits and vegetables, including grapes, varies widely from subspecies to subspecies, according to the species' individual phenolic composition. Additionally, antioxidant activity among varieties within a subspecies may vary, too, as a result of growth conditions—the amount of moisture the plant receives, the amount of sunlight it gets, the altitude at which it grows, the changes in temperature it experiences during growth, the concentration of insects in the area, the species of insects in the area, the season of harvest, and other factors. Therefore, high phenolic content, though indicative of antioxidant activity, is not necessarily analogous to high antioxidant activity.[2,23,24]

To my knowledge, only one scientific study has compared the antioxidant activities of Georgian wines to the antioxidant activities of non-Georgian wines. In this study, wines of the European Union nation Spain were examined. Researchers found that the average phenolic content of the Georgian wines was 1.83 times greater than the phenolic content of the Spanish wines. And even more important, they found that the average antioxidant activity of the Georgian wines was 1.59 times greater than that of the Spanish wines.[25] As you will read, traditional Georgians had access to far greater amounts of antioxidant phenolics from other plant sources. However, the high amounts of beneficial phenolics in Georgian wines did add to the tremendous total amount of healthful phenolics and other nutrients which were available through traditional Georgian foods and drinks.

HERBAL TEA

American adults drink an average 1.72 cups of coffee per day.[26,27,28] Often instead of coffee, traditional Georgians also regularly drank a few unique, highly nutritionally beneficial, naturally caffeine-free teas.

The most beloved of all Georgian teas was alpine tea, which was consumed after nearly every meal (and especially after fatty meals). Alpine tea was made from the leaves of *Rhododendron caucasicum*, a plant Georgians considered to be both a symbol of their country and a symbol of their longevity. Over the centuries, Georgians recognized alpine tea's effectiveness at treating a number of adverse health conditions.

When someone became ill, the usual first course of action was to administer alpine tea or to increase the patient's consumption of alpine tea twofold or threefold. Improvements in health usually followed and were often dramatic.[2]

The fact is, *Rhododendron caucasicum* contains some of the most powerful free radical neutralizers—substances that repair damaging, electron-deficient molecules—known to date. Among other things, modern research has shown that *Rhododendron caucasicum* extract can do the following:

- Protect against, and treat, heart dysfunction, artery damage, and lung damage
- Help normalize blood pressure, pulse rate, and cholesterol levels
- Help prevent degeneration of the brain and eyes
- Slow the progression of arthritis
- Prevent and treat gout
- Reduce the absorption of fat
- Stimulate the break-up of stored fat
- Strengthen blood vessels
- Protect and detoxify the liver
- Increase the availability of vitamin E in blood
- Inhibit the activity of viruses and pathogenic bacteria[29-41]

Clearly, consuming tea made from this *Rhododendron caucasicum* would have a tremendous affect on a person's health and well-being.

Another unique Georgian tea was made from flavorful Caucasian blueberry leaves. Among other positive activities, these leaves have been shown to do the following:

- Reduce glucose, LDL (bad cholesterol), and triglyceride levels

- Help protect against heart dysfunction and damage caused by nitrites
- Help prevent stomach cancers and brain degeneration
- Help prevent damage caused by pesticides and radiation
- Inhibit viral activity, among other benefits[41-53]

So again, simply by regularly drinking tea made with Caucasian blueberry leaves, traditional Georgians would have protected their health and ensured their longevity.

Finally, many traditional Georgians also frequently drank tea made from the root of the plant *Rhodiola rosea*. Among other benefits, this plant has been shown to do the following:

- Effectively prevent and treat depression, stress, and stress-related disorders
- Improve mental performance, including memory
- Improve physical performance, including sexual performance
- Improve hearing
- Stimulate the break-up of stored fat
- Protect and detoxify the liver
- Increase the body's resistance to the harmful effects of too little oxygen, too much oxygen, radiation, toxins, cold, and strenuous exercise[53-67]

Clearly, with so many benefits, teas made from *Rhodiola rosea* and the other plants were very important to the success of the Georgian diet. And because they were so important to ensuring Georgian health and longevity, the plants from which these teas were made will be discussed in more detail in the chapters to come.

POMEGRANATE FRUIT, JUICE AND SEEDS

Large salads were part of every traditional Georgian meal, and these salads were composed of the nutrient-dense leaves and berries of a variety of plants, along with ground walnuts and horse chestnuts. Also important were the salad dressings Georgians ate with their salads. These dressings were made from yogurt mixed with the juice and seeds of pomegranate, to which a variety of other fruit and vegetable juices were added to produce unique flavors. That base of pomegranate seeds and juice turns out to be very important to ensuring good health.

Research now shows that Georgian pomegranate can, among other things, do the following:

- Protect against DNA damage
- Kill cancer cells, inhibit the development and reproduction of cancer cells, and inhibit the number of cancerous tumors
- Help prevent the oxidation of cholesterol
- Reduce the absorption of LDL (bad cholesterol) by arterial cells
- Reduce the size of atherosclerotic lesions—areas where cholesterol has built up in the arteries and hardened
- Inhibit pathogenic bacteria[68-77]

And since pomegranate is a very popular fruit in Georgia and traditional Georgians ate pomegranate apples, drank pomegranate juice, and also basted meats with sauces made from Georgian pomegranate,[2] it is clear that these people's health and longevity was positively influenced by the fruit. That is why, along with the three plants just mentioned, Georgian pomegranate will also be discussed in more detail in a subsequent chapter.

GLACIAL MILK

Throughout history, Georgians have been drinking slightly gray water that is relatively thick and slippery. This water is known around the world as *glacial milk, slippery water*, or *gray water*. I will refer to it as *glacial milk*.

As the glaciers of the Caucasus Mountains melt, mineral-rich runoff water weaves its way through ancient, eroded tunnels and channels, collecting additional mineral dust. Eventually, it drains into aquifers that supply Georgia's thousands of wells and natural springs. The more than five hundred different glacial milk varieties that come from these wells and springs are known by specific names that relate to the places they're bottled. Some of these varieties include Borjomi, Sairme, Nabeglavi, Zvare, Java, and Kugela.[78,79,80] Today this water is bottled and sold in markets. However, traditional Georgians would often travel miles to get glacial milk, preferably directly from a spring or a well.[2,81]

Glacial milk has several benefits. Its unique appearance, taste, and "thickness" are due, in part, to its unusually high concentration of minerals, and innumerable studies have already demonstrated that minerals are essential to every function of the human body. Besides that, many minerals have antioxidant activity. Additionally, Georgian glacial milk contains bicarbonates that assist in maintaining healthy pH.[2] Among other benefits, maintaining a proper pH balance supports the growth of healthy microflora in the intestines, and maintaining a healthy environment in the intestines is in turn a prerequisite to good health and longevity.[82,83,84] Of course, glacial milk in not chlorinated; drinking chlorinated water damages the microflora of the intestines and has been implicated in other health disorders.[2,85,86]

An analysis of the Georgian glacial milk called *Borjomi*

reveals that this water's slipperiness is caused primarily by its high volume of bicarbonates. The low friction of this slippery water allows it to flow more easily through the body, among other things. Consequently, glacial milk is extremely effective at hydrating the body, delivering nutrients to all parts of the body, effectively rinsing the body, and aiding in the release of toxins from the body.[2] Clearly, drinking such water helped traditional Georgians stay healthy.

MATZONI AND KEFIR

Traditional Georgians, like many Caucasian peoples, regularly consumed tremendous amounts of probiotic-rich foods, especially specific yogurts called matzoni and kefir. But before we can discuss these foods and their benefits, an explanation of probiotics is necessary.

Each person's approximately twenty-seven feet of intestines contains trillions of living microorganisms. Among these are about four hundred to five hundred species of bacteria, many of which are bad for us, but most of which are good. The good bacteria in our intestines are known as probiotics. In the large intestines alone, where most bacterial activity occurs, this microbial mix—the intestinal flora—accounts for about 30 percent (and as much as 50 percent) of the colon's contents.[87-92]

Probiotics are essential to good health and have many functions. They form a lubricating film which helps protect the walls of the intestines from friction and scrape damage, and from attachment and invasion by pathogens—harmful, disease-producing substances. Probiotics also help break down foods, thereby preparing nutrients for absorption. They assist in passing food through the intestines. This helps prevent constipation and it moves harmful substances out of the body before they can be absorbed into the bloodstream. Finally, probiotics compete with bad bacteria and other microorganisms for nutrients, thereby suppressing populations of pathogens that otherwise could degrade good health and put stress on the immune system. These good bacteria have even been used to treat several health disorders.[89-106]

Unfortunately, as we grow older, pathogenic (bad) bacteria progressively displace probiotics (good bacteria) in our intestines.[106,107] This displacement can be exacerbated by illnesses or surgeries.[93] In addition, stress, natural and pharmaceutical antibiotics, birth-control pills, aspirin, alcohol, sugar, high fat and high meat diets, antibacterial chemicals, radiation, chlorine, laxatives, and antacids can all kill, retard, or displace the probiotics we must maintain in our systems.[95] These problems are compounded by the fact that the foods we consume today contain fewer probiotics than ever before.[96]

There are only two solutions to maintaining a healthy amount of probiotics in our systems. First, when possible, we can avoid substances that are harmful to probiotics. Second, we can consume high quality, live probiotics either through the foods we eat or through nutritional supplements. This is where the traditional Georgian diet comes in.

One of the world's most probiotic-rich foods is matzoni, which is similar in appearance, taste, and content to its sister yogurt, kefir. Matzoni was developed by people of the Caucasus Mountains area, and it was a staple of the Georgian diet for more than two thousand years. Until recently, it was consumed during nearly every Georgian meal.[2] In fact, as Sula Benet explains, "in western Georgia, an area where the greatest percentage of centenarians reside, over two pounds of probiotic-rich matzoni and other dairy products were consumed daily per capita."[81]

The base ingredient in matzoni is cow, goat, sheep, ewe, horse, or buffalo milk. Several species of probiotics and beneficial yeasts are added to the milk, and the formulation is allowed to ferment. The end result is a probiotic-rich yogurt that has more of a liquid consistency than most other yogurts.

Matzoni is very easy to digest, and it also aids in the digestion of other foods. Therefore, it is a sensible counterpart to heavy food. It is also an excellent choice for babies, the elderly, those with digestive disorders, and those who wish to prevent digestive disorders.[2,81]

The health benefits of any yogurt depend on the amounts and species of probiotics the yogurt contains. Because of their probiotics, matzoni and kefir are far more biologically active and medicinally potent than American-style yogurts. Typical American yogurts, for example, contain just two species of probiotics from two genera, whereas various matzonis and kefirs normally contain between ten and twenty species of probiotics from six to ten genera.[108,109,110] However, even these much less potent American yogurts usually accomplish at least the minimum of their prescribed duties quite effectively. In many countries, including the United States, an increasing number of physicians recommend yogurts to patients whose intestinal flora (probiotic volume) has been temporarily wiped out by antibiotics.

In eating matzoni, traditional Georgians benefited from more than just the probiotics. This is because of the way in which many Georgians ate this special yogurt. Because the taste of undiluted *Rhododendron caucasicum* is quite bitter, some two thousand years ago Georgians discovered they could hide the bitterness by mixing into it matzoni and kefir.[2,110,111] In addition to providing a more palatable way to consume *Rhododendron caucasicum*, it provided a welcome side benefit. It further fortified kefir and matzoni's antipathogenic activities and thereby allowed the yogurts to last longer before turning rancid.[2]

In addition to using this plant with matzoni and kefir, Georgians began baking *Rhododendron caucasicum* breads and brewing *Rhododendron caucasicum* tea, which became known throughout the region as alpine tea.[2,29,30] Of course, as has been previously discussed, this tea also provided many health benefits.

The Georgian Diet and Nutrition Today

Today, the validity of traditional Georgian dietary practices is finally being recognized. (It is interesting that Georgian ideas about nutrition and exercise are now treated as seemingly modern discoveries by Western and other non-Georgian scientists.) A simple search in the National Library of Medicine reveals more than 100,000 studies performed during the last thirty years that correlate diet to preventing disease or slowing its onset. And another 100,000 studies performed during the last thirty years show how exercise affects health.[112]

Despite this research, however, good health and nutrition still haven't fully entered the general American consciousness. Only 32 of 125 U.S. medical schools required their students to take a course in nutrition as of 1997.[113] And regardless of the research, much of which has been publicized by mainstream media, Americans continue to consume an increasingly high volume of calories—often from unhealthy foods—as part of their diets. In 1978, American adults consumed an average 1,969 calories per day, and by the year 2000, the average American caloric intake had increased to 2,200 calories per day. This high caloric intake continues today. Many of the calories are empty, originating in soft drinks and heavily processed foods that have little or no nutritional value. At the same time, the Centers for Disease Control and Prevention in Atlanta report that more than 60 percent of American adults are inactive, rarely performing any physical activity. This comes as officials at the National Heart, Lung, and Blood Institute say that even a brisk, thirty-minute walk each day can make a big difference in a person's weight and health.[114-117]

In deep contrast, adherents to the traditional Georgian diet typically consumed between 1,500 and 1,700 calories a day.[118] Besides that, most of the calories traditional Georgians consumed were derived from fresh, nutrient-rich foods. Certainly, traditional Georgians were not completely without a few bad habits, including a love for barbecued foods. But in spite of such factors, the tremendous healthy longevity of the Georgian centenarians remained.[2]

Now, I believe, based on the preponderance of research, that the low-calorie, nutrient-dense drinks and fresh foods that traditional Georgians regularly consumed played a major role in helping to protect these people from disease. This diet promoted good physical and mental health and activity, and thereby advanced longevity.

I've explained some of the basics of the traditional Georgian diet already, and in the book's remaining chapters, I will explore several of the most important elements of the diet in much greater detail. These elements include the four amazingly beneficial plants: *Rhododendron caucasicum*, Caucasian blueberry leaves, Georgian pomegranate, and *Rhodiola rosea*.

CHAPTER 3

Rhododendron Caucasicum

Traditional Georgians have long believed there is a correlation between the consumption of alpine tea, which is made from *Rhododendron caucasicum*, and overall good health, well being, and longevity. An abundance of modern research has subsequently confirmed *Rhododendron caucasicum*'s tremendous medicinal and nutritional properties. For example, scientists who have performed or studied *Rhododendron caucasicum* now realize that drinking tea made from this plant after meals—particularly after fatty meals—or consuming *Rhododendron caucasicum* by other means before meals helps our bodies to eliminate saturated animal fat, maintain optimum weight, and in several additional ways promote longevity. For these reasons, I will present *Rhododendron caucasicum* first of four of the most important plant species regularly consumed by long-living Georgians.

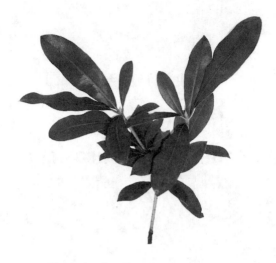

Rhododendron caucasicum spring leaves

Rhododendron Caucasicum: An Introduction

First, here are some basic facts about rhododendrons. Rhododendron is one of the largest and most diverse genera in the plant kingdom. The genus consists of more than 850 species and many thousands of varieties. Today, rhododendrons are widely distributed and have been found on all of earth's continents except Africa and South America. Five species of rhododendron grow in the republic of Georgia, all of which have been used in varying degrees in folk medicines. Of these five species, extracts of three are used for the same purposes in certain conventional medicines. These three extracts, of which one is produced from *Rhododedron caucasicum*, generally are refered to as rhododendron extracts. The name rhododendron is derived from the Greek *rhodon*, meaning "rose," and *dendron*, meaning "tree."[1-7]

The most important of all species of rhododendron is *Rhododendron caucasicum*.[2,5] This species has been best described by the renowned Russian scientist Musa Abidoff, M.D., who wrote the following: "The species *Rhododendron caucasicum* (Caucasian snow rose/high altitude snow rose) is an evergreen bush [that] grows at altitudes of...[5,200 to 10,000[5]] feet high on the Caucasian Mountains in the northern region of the republic of Georgia. *Rhododendron caucasicum*, indigenous to the Caucasian Mountains . . . possesses various health-promoting properties."[9] It is also one of the very few species of rhododendron that has proven safe for human consumption.[1,2,5,8,9]

"In Georgian traditional medicine," Dr. Abidoff continues, "the *Rhododendron caucasicum* remedy was used for coughs, removing phlegm, and chronic bronchitis, and it was used in the treatment of arthritis and gout. It also was used for myalgic (muscle) pains whether rheumatic or not, but especially of the facial and eye regions. Tea of *Rhododendron caucasicum*'s spring leaves and buds also [has] been used in [treating] glaucoma, heart irregularities, depression, burst blood vessels in the eyes, bacterial and viral infections, etc."[9]

Research History of Rhododendron

Georgian-grown species of rhododendron first became a subject of modern scientific investigations during the early 1900s. By late 1932 scientists found that the leaves of the species *Rhododendron caucasicum* contained an unusually high volume of phenolics.[2,5,10] This discovery prompted further research into the biochemistry and metabolism of *Rhododendron caucasicum* and other species of rhododendrons found in the republic of Georgia. Georgian research on these rhododendrons continued throughout the early 1940s, but it wasn't until after World War II that research on the plants intensified. Beginning during the late 1940s, Georgian and Russian scientists conducted pharmacological research on both the plants and their constituents. Also, the toxicity levels of the plant's constituents and extracts were researched and identified, and various studies determined the plant's optimum harvest times and the best methods of extracting, concentrating, and standardizing rhododendron's most beneficial chemicals.

By late 1952, clinical studies were underway in Russia to measure the effectiveness of rhododendron-based extracts in treating several diseases.[5,11-18] Then, in 1954, after these and other research results had been analyzed, the U.S.S.R. Health Department recommended rhododendron-based extracts for the treatment of high blood pressure, retinal hemorrhages, circulatory insufficiency, and chronic venous insufficiency, or failure of a deteriorated blood-return system to sufficiently remove waste from tissues.[1,2,8,19] These were the first of many officially recommended medicinal applications for *Rhododendron caucasicum*.

Also during the 1940s and 1950s, research on *Rhododendron caucasicum* got another boost. This came primarily through the work of Albert Szent-Gyorgyi von Nagyrapolt, M.D., Ph.D., the Hungarian scientist who decades earlier had discovered, characterized, and named vitamin C—an accomplishment that earned him the 1937 Nobel Prize in physiology/medicine. While researching vitamin C, Dr. Szent-Gyorgyi discovered, characterized, and named P-vitamin activity, which became important in *Rhododendron caucasicum* research.[20-25]

Here is a little background information about P-vitamins: The word "P-vitamin" actually represents a group of nutrients, each of which is a phenolic and each of which is a flavonoid. Stated in more detail, some phytochemicals (plant

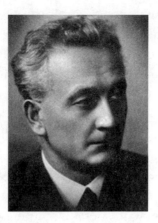

Albert Szent-Gyorgyi, M.D., Ph.D., the Hungarian scientist
who discovered and characterized vitamin C and
P-vitamin (specific flavonoid) activity

chemicals) are phenolics, some phenolics are flavonoids
and/or phenolic acids, all flavonoids exhibit P-vitamin activity, and all P-vitamins are flavonoids. In addition, all flavonoids
are antioxidants, or free radical neutralizers. P-vitamins help
the body in many ways, including:

• Their presence allows vitamin C to be properly absorbed
and processed.

• Their individual antioxidant properties provide myriad
health benefits, including protection against capillary
fragility. Examples of capillary fragility include heart disease, strokes (in which blood vessels of the brain become
weak and burst), varicose veins, hemorrhoids, bloody noses,
and bleeding gums.[2,5,8,20,25]

Dr. Albert Szent-Gyorgyi's revolutionary discovery of P-
vitamin activity had created massive scientific interest in

Georgia, but subsequent research on the subject was tremendously inhibited by World War II. However, by the early 1950s, studies of flavonoid-rich plants, which naturally exhibit P-vitamin activity, became a top priority for a few scientists at Georgia's Tblisi State University. One of those scientists was professor Sergei Vasil'evich Durmishidze, Ph.D., who had founded the university's Department of Plant Biochemistry and who later founded the Georgian Academy of Science's Institute of Plant Biochemistry.[2,5,8,27,28] Professor Durmishidze and his colleagues demonstrated that many of *Rhododendron caucasicum*'s medicinal properties came because the plant exhibited significant P-vitamin activity.[2,5,27] They also confirmed the fact that the constituents in *Rhododendron caucasicum* that are most responsible for the plant's pharmacological activity are a group of special phenolic acids and flavonoids.[2,5,8,9,20] This confirmed that many of *Rhododendron*

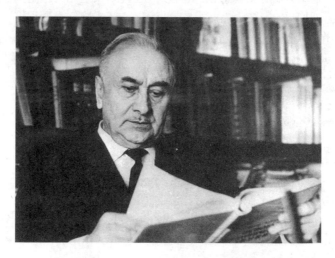

Professor Sergei Vasil'evich Durmishidze, Ph.D., the renown Georgian plant biochemist. Dr. Durmishidze produced a wealth of research on flavonoids and the P-vitamin activity of Georgian medicinal plants, including *Rhododendron caucasicum*.

caucasicum's medicinal properties came because the plant exhibited significant P-vitamin activity.

All of this activity was underway decades before the American scientific community recognized the tremendous importance of phytochemicals, phenolic acids, flavonoids, or P-vitamin activity.[8,26] As the American medical doctor Timothy J. Smith wrote in his book *Renewal: The Anti-Aging Revolution*, "It wasn't until the late 1980s that the enormous number and biological complexity of phytochemicals became evident. When nutritionally blasé molecular biologists realized that phytochemicals could also act as antioxidants, they suddenly got very excited . . . And when those same scientists began seeing the intimate connection between antioxidant phytochemicals and cellular protection, repair, and regeneration, they suddenly got religion."[26]

Georgian research on the properties of that country's medicinal plants continued throughout the remainder of the twentieth century and is still being conducted today.[5,6,28-31] Three further developments in *Rhododendron caucasicum* research deserve special notes, however. During 1969, German Drs. H. Thieme, E. Walewska and H. J. Winkler reported the discovery of the beneficial compound salidroside in rhododendron, and Georgian scientists later confirmed its presence in *Rhododendron caucasicum*.[8,32] Salidroside is an adaptogen—a substance that helps the body adapt to and manage physical and psychological stresses. Salidroside is believed to be especially effective in improving function of the cardiovascular system, and in increasing blood supply to the muscles and the brain.[8,33,34] And during 1981, Georgian Drs. S. V. Durmishidze, A. G. Shalashvilee, V. V. Mzhavandadze and G. C. Tsiklauree published their laboratory research on rhododendrons, as well as analysis of other research on rhododendrons spanning over eighty years from around the world. Their findings confirmed the superiority of two species of rhododendon, both of which grow in the republic of Georgia, both of which have been used in Georgian folk and conventional medicines, and one of which is *Rhododendron caucasicum*. Of the two superior species, however, *Rhododendron caucasicum*'s medicinal preeminence again became apparent. UV-spectroscopy method analysis and chromatographic method analysis showed that *Rhododendron caucasicum* leaves contain well over twice the amount of flavonoids, including special and highly functional flavonoids, than those of the other species.[5] This confirmed that *Rhododendron caucasicum* has far greater P-vitamin activity and antioxidant potential than the other species. And finally, during 1997, the Georgian-born, Russian-American scientist Zakir Ramazanov, Ph.D.—the scientist who introduced me to *Rhododendron caucasicum*—reported that researchers had recently discovered another important phytochemical in the plant. This phytochemical was dihydroflavonol, called taxifolin and its glycoside astilbin (taxifolin + astilbin = dihydroflavonol)—or, to reiterate, a flavonoid that is among the most beneficial of all phenolics.[2,8,35] The presence of taxifolins is very rare in the plant kingdom,[2] so this was another particularly significant discovery. It helped further explain why *Rhododendron caucasicum* is adept at preventing and treating an array of illnesses.

Before discussing the plant's use in treating specific illnesses, however, we need a little more background into one of the chemical activities that makes *Rhododendron caucasicum* effective. Specifically, we need to further explore the concept of free radicals and free radical neutralizers—which all flavonoids are—to understand where much of *Rhododendron caucasicum*'s medicinal strength originates.

A Free-Radical Neutralizer

The concept of free radicals has been mentioned several times at this point, but without an intensive description of this enemy. However, understanding free radicals is crucial to understanding *Rhododendron caucasicum*. The fact is, much of *Rhododendron caucasicum*'s strength lies in its ability to neutralize free radicals in the body. This ability accounts for much of what allows the plant to prevent and treat diseases.

So what exactly are free radicals? We've previously described them as unstable molecules, each of which are missing an electron, and that damage other molecules in the body because of it. But let's step back even further to explain how stable molecules become unstable.

The human body is constantly barraged by toxins and other agents that interact with its cells in potentially negative ways. These agents enter the body through various actions, including touch, breathing, eating, and poor digestion. Generally, when one of these agents—a toxin, for example—reaches a cell in the human body, it damages the architecture of the cell's molecules, leaving behind one or more molecules with unpaired electrons. Any event that causes a molecule to gain too much oxygen, lose too much hydrogen, or otherwise lose electrons is referred to as oxidation. The remaining oxidized molecule with one or more unpaired electrons is referred to as a free radical.

Upon becoming free radicals, most unstable molecules react by immediately attempting to steal replacement electrons from other molecules. If this action is not neutralized, the free radicals can create an exponentially growing chain reaction of damage to other molecules, wherein hundreds, thousands, millions, or even billions of additional molecules become free radicals, sometimes within a billionth of a sec-

ond. Because cells are composed of molecules, every molecule of a cell that is damaged means that the cell is damaged.
As a result, the damaged cell begins to fail at what it was
designed to do.

Oxidation or free radical damage is part of our existence.
Stress causes it, as does exercise. But then again, so does
breathing, because oxygen—the very substance we need to
live—is itself a free radical and is among the most common
oxidizing agents. The most severe free radical damage, however, is caused by toxins—tobacco smoke, industrial pollutants, food additives, insecticides, and so on. We instinctively
seem to know that these toxins are bad for us.

In recent years, free radical damage has been connected
with a variety of specific bodily ills. Free radicals have been
shown to damage vital components and membranes of cells,
which leads to changes in the structure and function of the
cells. A free radical cascade can become excessive and cause
heart disease, strokes, tumors, cancer, emphysema,
Alzheimer's disease, Parkinson's disease, cataracts, rheumatoid arthritis, and other diseases. In other words, we are aging
and dying because of free radical damage.

Research has shown that natural substances called antioxidants or free radical neutralizers can repair cellular free radicals. Natural free radical neutralizers do this by donating one
of their own electrons or a hydrogen atom to the cellular free
radical. After the free radical neutralizer has repaired the free
radical, it becomes a free radical itself. However, it is less reactive than a typical free radical, and it is able to repair itself by
interacting with other free radical neutralizers.[36-44]

Because free radical damage has been implicated in many
diseases,[45] it is possible that free radical neutralizers may help
in preventing or even curing those diseases. It therefore
makes sense to maintain effective free radical neutralizers in

our systems to constantly slow and repair the molecular destruction caused by free radicals. That is where *Rhododendron caucasicum* comes in. *Rhododendron caucasicum* contains some of the most powerful free radical neutralizers, or antioxidants, known to date. These include hydroxycinnamic, chlorogenic, and gallic acid derivatives and taxifolins.[46,47,48]

Today, the positive impact of *Rhododendron caucasicum*'s powerful antioxidants is increasingly being demonstrated in scientific research. The plant has been shown to help prevent and treat numerous illnesses and conditions, and its medicinal potential is just beginning to be realized.

Health Solutions

The illnesses and health conditions *Rhododendron caucasicum* can help prevent and treat range from atherosclerosis (hardening of the arteries with plaque buildup on the interior arterial walls) to glaucoma and from gout to obesity. For much of the rest of the chapter, we'll explore these illnesses and *Rhododendron caucasicum*'s use in combating them.

OBESITY

More than half of the adult population in the United States is now overweight, and in recent years, the number of overweight people has risen dramatically. Between 1960 and 1994, the prevalence of overweight American adults increased from 31.6 percent of the population to 32.6 percent. But by 2000, 57.3 percent of the adult population was overweight, and by 2002, this number had grown to 61 percent. Also by 2002, the prevalence of obese adult Americans, or those who are extremely overweight, had grown to well over 25 percent of the population.[49-52] The fact is, the total number of overweight and obese people has been increasing in every state of the United States. The condition affects both genders, all races, ethnicities, age groups, and educational levels, and both smokers and nonsmokers alike.[51,53,54]

The increase in childhood obesity is particularly frightening. During the 1970s, about 7 percent of American children were overweight or obese, but by 1991, the figure had increased to 11 percent.[55] Even more tragic, by 1998, 20 percent of American children were overweight or obese, and that percentage has continued to rise. Much of the problem is due to poor eating habits and a lack of exercise. This is particularly tragic because childhood is when habits are formed for a lifetime, so these children will likely continue to eat poorly and miss exercise throughout their lives.[56]

The statistics are also disgraceful and alarming when one considers that, because of weight-control issues, permanent damage is being done to these children's health at an early age. This damage has been discovered during scientific studies. For example, Dr. Emily Liu of Kaleida Health's Women's and Children's Hospital in Buffalo, New York, found that 13 percent of the 147 obese children she studied showed signs of fatty liver disease. This can lead to cirrhosis of the liver. [57,58] Also, a Yale University study tested the health of 167 obese children who were between four and eighteen years of age. Researchers found that 25 percent of the 55 children aged four to ten and 21 percent of the 112 children aged eleven to eighteen had impaired glucose tolerance and insulin insensitivity. Four percent of the tested adolescents were already victims of Type 2, or adult-onset, diabetes.[59]

Obviously, being overweight or obese can cause a host of problems and can increase the severity of nearly all adverse health conditions. Most notably, overweight and obese people of any age are at exceptionally high risk of developing diabetes. Simply being overweight, regardless of diet, decreases insulin sensitivity, and decreased insulin sensitivity results in high insulin levels and high glucose levels in the blood. Both of these conditions, in turn, speed aging and can result in early death. Furthermore, prolonged high levels of insulin cause the liver to release excessive amounts of triglycerides, thereby flooding our systems with even more dangerous fat.[60-64]

But diabetes-related diseases are only one example of the myriad adverse health conditions that disproportionately afflict those who are overweight or obese. Research has revealed many more. For instance, according to the U.S. Centers for Disease Control and Prevention, the number of Americans diagnosed with high blood pressure increased by almost 10 percent between 1991 and 1999, and CDC researchers suspect the increase may be linked to the increases in overweight or obese Americans.[65] Then on January 16, 2002, the CDC reported that as many as 47 million Americans, or over 17.5 percent of the U.S. population, may be victims of a recently discovered, weight-related syndrome. This syndrome manifests itself in a combination of obesity, abdominal fat, insulin resistance, high blood glucose levels, high triglyceride levels, high cholesterol, and high blood pressure. It is also associated with nonalcoholic fatty liver disease and polycystic ovary syndrome, the symptoms of which are infertility, excess facial hair, and obesity in women.[66,67,68] During late August 2002, the American Association of Clinical Endocrinologists reported that further research indicates 33 percent of Americans may now be suffering from the syndrome.[67,68]

Weight also appears to be related to cancer. A study performed on 89,000 nurses, for example, found that those who rarely exercised, who were overweight, and who ate a lot of starchy foods, such as potatoes and white bread, more than doubled their risk of developing pancreatic cancer.[63,69] Medical research has also linked excess weight to cancers of the breast, uterus, colon, rectum, kidney, esophagus, gall bladder, cervix, ovaries, liver, stomach, and prostate, and to myeloma and non-Hodgkin's lymphoma. Notably, on April 24, 2003, the results of a sixteen-year study on 900,000 people were revealed. Researchers found that excess weight probably accounts for 14 percent of all male cancer deaths and 20 percent of all female cancer deaths.[70] Commenting on the study, Dr. Donna Ryan, head of clinical research at the Pennington Biomedical Research Center in Baton Rouge, Louisiana, told the Associated Press, "Because of the magnitude and strength of the study, it's irrefutable. It's absolutely convincing. And therefore it's frightening."[71]

Excess weight also affects pregnancy. Another study by the Centers for Disease Control and Prevention found that women who were obese or overweight during pregnancy were twice as likely to have babies with heart defects or multiple birth defects. Furthermore, obese women were three times as likely as women of normal weight to give birth to babies suffering from omphalocele, a condition in which intestines or other abdominal organs protrude through the navel.[72,73]

The cost of treatment for weight-related illnesses, premature death, and lost wages and productivity due to being overweight is estimated to be as high as $117 billion dollars per year in the United States alone—and the economic and medical toll of the illnesses continue to increase. On August 30, 2002, the CDC estimated that excess weight and obesity result in more than 300,000 premature American deaths per year.[74,75]

Clearly, obesity and poor weight control have become two of the most common and dangerous disorders of the twenty-first century. I believe they are, at least partially, the result of rapid economic evolution and the inability of our bodies to keep pace.

Programmed weight retention. Since the beginning of human history, our species has evolved in circumstances where nutrients were in short supply. One never knew if the next meal would be found in an hour, a day, a week, or longer. In order for humanity to survive, our bodies developed physiological methods to combat weight loss and retain energy stores. But these natural methods of self-preservation have resulted in obesity when coupled with modern societal eating habits.

As recently as the 1940s, before and during World War II, many young American military recruits, especially from rural areas, were so malnourished that they failed their enlistment physicals.[76] Interestingly, during the fifty-plus years since the end of World War II—a mere blink of the eye in evolutionary terms—we have burst forth into an age of superabundance. Suddenly, big portions of tasty, varied foods are available everywhere, and at reasonable prices.[77]

The problem with this new age of abundance is that our bodies are still programmed to collect and store fat to protect our organs from nutrient depletion. The bigger we become, the more provisions our bodies attempt to maintain. In other words, being overweight forces us to eat more and more. This natural phenomenon and a lack of daily physical activity slow the process of eliminating unwanted pounds. And the more inactive we become, the more easily we become fatigued, depressed, and lethargic—conditions that further reduce any motivation we have to exercise. This is compounded by the fact that when we do diet, the body, to protect its existence, slows its release of energy, thereby creating even more fatigue, depression, and lethargy. All of this leads to further weight retention.

The good news is that there is a solution, and it lies in blocking fat absorption.

Fat absorption. The average Westerner consumes about 100 grams of fat per day. About 95 percent of that fat consists of triglycerides. These triglycerides must be broken down before they can be absorbed through the intestinal membranes.

The enzyme responsible for breaking down triglycerides and making the fats available for absorption is called pancreatic lipase. This enzyme is found in the gastrointestinal tract. It binds to the surface of the intestinal wall, which comes in contact with food. When pancreatic lipase is absent, dietary fats are not absorbed. Instead, these fats are excreted.

Of course, our bodies need some fat in order to perform properly. Consider these facts:

- About 40 percent of the energy we use is provided by fat.
- Fats are the primary building blocks of cell membranes.
- Fats are the only source of essential fatty acids.
- Fats are necessary for the processing and uptake of vitamins A, D, E and K.

However, research indicates that the amount of fat most Americans consume can, and probably should, be dramatically reduced. Therefore, if a safe and natural method to *partially* block pancreatic lipase activity could be found, it would provide a much desired way to easily reduce the amount of fat that is absorbed from the diet.[2,78-84]

Blocking fat absorption. Western pharmaceutical companies recently introduced a new class of lipase-inhibiting drugs—drugs commonly referred to as fat blockers—but recent scientific studies have revealed that Georgians have been limiting their fat absorption for many centuries. They've been doing so with the natural pancreatic lipase inhibitor: *Rhododendron caucasicum*.

As previously described, traditional Georgians have been consuming *Rhododendron caucasicum* spring leaves since before the time of Christ.[2,8,20] Those same natural and safe *Rhododendron caucasicum* spring leaves were recently found to be an effective pancreatic lipase inhibitor in clinical research done by professor Musa Abidoff, M.D., of the Moscow Center for Modern Medicine.[35,85]

In Dr. Abidoff's study, two types of rhododendron extracts were used as test medicines. These two types differed in their base plants' season of harvest; one extract came from *Rhododendron caucasicum* spring leaves, the other from *Rhododendron caucasicum* summer-fall leaves. One hundred thirty-two patients at Moscow State Hospital and Center for Modern Medicine were given 150 milligrams of one or the other type of rhododendron extract three times per day prior to food intake. Samples of their feces were then collected and analyzed for total fat and protein. At the same time, a placebo control group received the same food, but without either of the extracts.

As it turned out, rhododendron extract made from *Rhododendron caucasicum* spring leaves stimulated the release of fat into the feces far better than the inferior summer-fall extract, and certainly better than the useless substances the placebo group received. Of course, an *increase* in the amount of fat excreted means a *decrease* in the amount of fat absorbed through intestinal membranes and stored in the body. The result is less weight gain and more weight loss. And in fact, that is exactly what happened in the clinical trial. During the study's first three months, the patients who received rhododendron extract made from *Rhododendron caucasicum* spring leaves extract reduced their original weight an average of between five and twenty pounds. (It is important to note that the weight reduction came without the use of any of the popular weight-loss substances found on the market today, many of which are potentially quite harmful.[86,87]) These test subjects also showed statistically significant improvements in their bodies' protein-to-fat ratios.[35,85]

In reviewing the results of this study, Dr. Zakir Ramazanov said, "Some people might think that a reduction of five to twenty pounds within the first three months is not enough. But according to research, fast weight loss is not healthy, and people who lose weight very quickly regain weight very quickly. It is therefore advisable to lose weight slowly, and to keep in mind that there are substantial health benefits to even modest weight loss."[2]

Dr. Ramazanov's conclusions have proved correct in additional medical studies. For example, Dr. Lynn Moore, an assistant professor of medicine at Boston University, reviewed the medical files of about four hundred people who participated in the Framingham Heart Study, which began in 1948. The participants between the ages of thirty and fifty who lost four or more pounds and kept that weight off for four years were 25 percent less likely to develop high blood pressure during the next forty years. Participants between fifty and sixty-five years of age who did the same were 30 percent less likely to develop high blood pressure. And participants who lost between eight and fifteen pounds and kept it off for four years cut their diabetes risk by 33 percent. "It's amazing, isn't it?" Dr. Moore told Reuters. "Even that modest amount of weight loss makes a big difference. That's an exciting health message."[88,89]

As Dr. Moore's research shows, keeping off any weight you do lose is as important as initially losing the weight. However, the best practice is not to gain weight in the first place, particularly for those who are entering their middle adult years. And that's where *Rhododendron caucasicum* comes in. Consuming this plant from an early age can help prevent excess weight gain, thanks to its natural fat-blocking properties.

Releasing stored fat. Beyond reducing the amount of fat absorbed into the body, *Rhododendron caucasicum* also stimulates the release of fat from adipose tissue—the so-called fat pads, where triglycerides are stored. Releasing fatty acids from adipose tissue allows them to be burned off, which also results in weight loss.

On average, about 21 percent of male body weight and 26 percent of female body weight is made up of fat—enough to allow the average human to survive for two to three months without food.[82] It is naturally very difficult to force this stored fat out of its tissue-efficient storage. However, Dr. Toshi Motoyashiki and colleagues at Fukuyama University recently demonstrated that taxifolins—one of the major compounds in *Rhododendron caucasicum* spring leaves extract—stimulate the release of fat from adipose tissue. These Japanese researchers found that the decomposition of fat in the fat pads was stimulated by taxifolins alone.[90,91]

Of these results, Dr. Ramazanov says: "It is interesting to note that in addition to burning calories, exercise stimulates adipose tissue fat release, too. Fatty acids released from adipose tissue circulate with blood flow and eventually enter into cells to produce energy. Once fatty acids are released from fat tissue, it is important to use them, by burning them off, as soon as possible. This can be done through simple exercise."[2]

Dr. Ramazanov recommends four actions for successful permanent weight control:

• Reduce the amount of fat in your diet.
• Consume *Rhododendron caucasicum* about fifteen minutes before every meal.
• Consume *Rhododendron caucasicum* about thirty minutes prior to exercise.
• Perform some type of exercise, even moderate walking, at least once every day.[2,8]

HEART DISEASE

The human heart is truly an amazing organ. Each day, its 100,000 rhythmic contractions pump about 1,835 gallons of blood through more 60,000 miles of blood vessels in the human body. Thus, it supplies body tissues with the oxygen and nutrients necessary to sustain life.[92,93,94] When this organ is damaged, however, the results are severe. Fortunately, there are ways to protect the heart from damage and treat damage when it occurs. One of those ways is to consume *Rhododendron caucasicum*.

For many centuries, *Rhododendron caucasicum* has been used in Georgian folk medicine to support healthy heart function and to prevent and treat adverse heart conditions. Now, medical research, specifically clinical trials in which rhododendron extract was administered to heart patients, indicates that rhododendron extract helps normalize heart function and blood chemistry and helps protect the heart from and repair damage caused by free radicals, high blood pressure, and other stresses. These positive benefits are the result of the plant's P-vitamin activity, high levels of potent antioxidants, and its adaptogenic properties.

For one thing, rhododendron extract has been shown to have a positive effect on atherosclerotic patients—those whose arteries are progressively degenerating, thickening, accumulating plaque, becoming less elastic, and restricting blood flow. Professor Dmitry M. Rossiisskiy, M.D., a meritorious science worker at the U.S.S.R. Medical Academy of Science, conducted a clinical study using rhododendron extract to treat patients with these conditions. The tests were performed at the First Moscow Central Hospital's Cardiovascular Health and Prophylactic Centers, and a total of seventy test subjects diagnosed with circulatory insufficiency and atherosclerosis, with primary damage to the aorta, coronary vessels and mitral valve were observed. All were administered 70–150 milligrams of rhododendron extract three times per day for a period of fifteen to thirty-five days. As a result, the patients' blood circulation increased, their breathing improved, their urination increased substantially, the buildup of fluid in the lungs and liver was eliminated, and their pulses slowed by ten to fifteen beats per minute. Furthermore, some of the patients experienced reductions in the sizes of their enlarged hearts and livers.[7]

In another study, this one also performed at the First Moscow Central Hospital, Drs. A. G. Gukasyan and A. Y. Ivanova examined thirty hospitalized patients between the ages of fifteen and fifty-two. Each of the patients was suffering from one or more types of heart disease and most were in extremely serious condition. Five of the patients had shown no response to other heart medications such as digitalis, diuretics, etc., and also were suffering from end-stage cirrhosis of the liver and other diseases. All thirty patients were administered 200 to 300 milligrams of rhododendron extract twice per day for two to four weeks or longer. As a result, eleven patients showed improvements, and ten patients showed substantial improvements. In these twenty-one patients, breathing improved and their pulses slowed. In some cases urination increased, the buildup of fluids in the lungs and other organs disappeared, the velocity of blood circulation increased, and their blood pressures decreased.[12]

As previously mentioned, rhododendron extract has been shown to improve the health of heart patients who suffer from mitral valve disease—those whose mitral valves are dysfunctional resulting in increased workload on the heart. Now we will describe mitral valve disease and rhododenron extracts' effectiveness in the treatment of this illness in more detail.

The mitral valve is the gateway through which oxygenated blood is pumped from the upper left chamber to the lower left chamber of the heart. From there the blood flows throughout the body, delivering oxygen to all cells.[95,96] When a person's mitral valve does not function properly, the normal flow of blood in the heart is disrupted. The resulting unusual blood turbulance can cause a unique hum, whoosh or clicking sound—a murmur that can be heard through a stethoscope.[97,98,99]

Mitral valve disease can include mitral valve stenosis, in which blood flow is restricted because the valve doesn't open widely enough; mitral valve regurgitation, in which blood backflows because the valve won't close tightly enough; mitral valve flail, in which one or both of the leaflets/doors of the valve dip back into the chamber from which it is pumping blood; and mitral valve prolapse, in which one or both flaps of the mitral valve bulge during each contraction. While each of these forms of mitral valve disease have specific causes, the progression of one mitral valve disease can cause or worsen another mitral valve disease. Furthermore, mitral valve disease can also be aggravated by coronary artery disease, heart attack, cardiomyopathy (heart muscle disease), and other disorders. People with

mitral valve disease also are extra vulnerable, especially following certain dental or surgical procedures, to bacterial endo-
carditis, a rare but potentially fatal infection of the mitral valve
and lining of the heart.[95,100-104]

During a normal lifespan, most people eventually will suffer from some form of mitral valve disease.[105] In young adults,
the most common form of mitral valve disease is mitral valve
prolapse (MVP), which scientists believe affects between 5
and 6 percent of the general population. While approximately 60 percent of people with MVP experience no symptoms
whatsoever, 40 percent suffer from mild to severe symptoms.
These can include arrhythmias (irregular heartbeat), tachy-
cardia (sudden rapid heartbeat), breathing difficulties, chest
pain, panic attacks, fatigue, weakness, and fainting.[101-111] The
most severe effects of any mitral valve disease, including
MVP, can include heart attack, stroke, and heart failure.[100,101]

The good news is that, as mentioned, rhododendron
extract has been shown to positively affect patients who suffer from mitral valve disease. In one scientific study performed at Moscow State Hospital, Drs. N. D. Abramova and
S. S. Galpern observed twenty-four men and thirty-six
women between the ages of eighteen and sixty-five who had
been diagnosed with heart disease. Most of the patients' heart
dysfuntion was the result of mitral valve disease with first to
second degree blood circulation insufficiency. These patients
were given 70 to 150 milligrams of rhododendron extract
two to four times per day. Professor Dmitry M. Rossiisskiy,
M.D., who supervised the study stated: "In all cases the usage
of the preparation [rhododendron extract] led to positive
results."[7] The study, published in the journal *Pharmacology
and Toxicology*, revealed that in patients who received the
rhododendron extract, blood circulation increased and the
buildup of stagnating blood due to blockage was eliminated

Additionally, the patients' breathing improved, their urination increased substantially, and the patients' pulses slowed by ten to fifteen beats per minute.[7]

And rhododendron extract has been shown to have a positive effect in treating patients who suffer from rheumatic heart disease/rheumatic heart valve damage. (Rheumatic heart disease is a condition that begins with a streptococcus infection, such as strep throat, that progressed into rheumatic fever with resulting inflammation of joints and damage to one or more of the heart's four valves: the tricuspid valve, the mitral valve, the pulmonary semilunar valve, and the aortic semilunar valve.) In a Russian study that examined this phenomenon, 80 rheumatic heart disease patients between the ages of 19 and 60 who had symptoms of cardiac insufficiency were observed at the First Moscow Central Hospital. Along with their usual antirheumatic treatments, the patients were given 130 milligrams of rhododendron extract three times per day for two to three weeks. As a result, the patients' general health improved, their blood pressures went down, and their heart functions stabilized.[2,13,112]

Finally, studies have demonstrated that key constituents of rhododendron extract reduce LDL (bad cholesterol) levels and protect LDL from oxidation. Reducing LDL levels and protecting LDL from oxidation are important factors in the prevention and treatment of cardiovascular diseases, as will be described in detail in following chapters.[113-116]

ARTHRITIS

Arthritis and rheumatism are among the most common chronic diseases in the United States. Nearly 70 million Americans currently have arthritis, and this number represents an increase in the estimated number of sufferers by 27.3

million since 1997.[117,118] Just what are these diseases? Well, according to the Arthritis Foundation, the term "arthritis" actually refers to more than 100 separate conditions. All of them can affect people's quality of life and deprive them of their physical and financial independence.[73] One class of arthritic diseases, musculoskeletal diseases such as osteoarthritis and rheumatoid arthritis, now costs the U.S. economy an estimated $83 billion per year in care, lost wages, and lost productivity.[117,118]

One of the most common types of arthritis is osteoarthritis, or degenerative joint disease. This disease is characterized by the gradual breakdown of cartilage, the material that covers the ends of bones at the joints and acts as a cushion between bones. With osteoarthritis, the cartilage becomes irritated and inflamed, degrades, and begins to wear unevenly. Over time, it roughens and pieces break away. This allows opposing bones to come in contact with and grind against each other with every movement, which causes pain and thereby restricts movement. Eventually, outgrowths of new bone form, which cause more pain and further restrict movement.[120,121,122]

Osteoarthritis can range from being very mild to being severe. It commonly occurs in middle-aged and older people, although research has shown it is not an inevitable part of aging.[2,123] Even so, the causes of osteoarthritis are unknown.

One theory about what causes arthritis is that the disease comes from the abnormal release of an enzyme called hyaluronidase. In their book *New Secrets of Effective Natural Stress and Weight Management Using Rhodiola Rosea and Rhododendron Caucasicum*, Drs. Zakir Ramazanov and Maria del Mar Bernal Suarez, who have researched this enzyme, explain how this might work. "Hyaluronidase is released from the cartilage cells, which leads to cartilage breakdown and destruction of the joint. Hyaluronidase breaks down the

Table 4. Inhibition of Hyaluronidase—Test 1

Hyaluronidase activity	Percentage of inhibition
Rhododendron extract	90
Grape seed extract	38
Pine bark extract	45

Source: Zakir Ramazanov, Ph.D. 1997, 1999. [124,125]

hyaluronic acid that is an essential constituent in collagen," they write. "Factors that influence the activity of this enzyme include diet, pH, and microbial ecology in the gut."[124] (And as Drs. Ramazanov and del Mar Bernal Suarez further note, besides its arthritic implications, this enzyme is also known to activate carcinogens that can lead to colon cancer.[124])

Fortunately for those concerned about arthritis, research shows that rhododendron extract is very active against hyaluronidase. Drs. Ramazanov and del Mar Bernal Suarez reported on this research, which was performed at the Georgian Institute of Plant Biochemistry. In the study, the hyaluronidase-inhibiting activity of rhododendron extract was compared with the activity of two other extracts, grape seed and pine bark. Like rhododendron extract, both grape seed extract and pine bark extract contain flavonoids and the extracts are often used by arthritis sufferers. In the end, the researchers found that rhododendron extract was much stronger at inhibiting hyaluronidase than either grape seed or pine bark extracts.

They even tested these results on arthritic rabbits and learned that with rhododendron extract, "the effect of hyaluronidase on skin collagen degradation was nearly abolished," while the other extracts' enzyme-inhibiting activity was significantly lower.[124]

GOUT

Gout affects about 2 million Americans—men much more often than women—and is one of the most painful diseases known to man.[126] It causes swelling, redness, heat, and stiffness in the joints, and sudden, severe attacks of pain. Though it can affect the knees, ankles, feet, hands, wrists, and elbows, gout usually affects one joint at a time and tends to manifest itself in a toe. A big toe affected with gout can become so sensitive that even a bed sheet brushing against it can produce an intense amount of pain.

The pain and swelling associated with gout are caused by a buildup of uric acid in an affected joint. Uric acid is waste product that normally forms when the body breaks down certain proteins. Ordinarily, uric acid is dissolved in the blood and passed through the kidneys and into the urine, where it is eliminated. However, if the body increases its production of uric acid and/or if the kidneys fail to eliminate enough uric acid, excess uric acid crystals can form in the soft tissues of the joints and cause gout. Additionally, uric acid crystals can appear as lumps under the skin near joints and at the rim of the ear. Uric acid crystals can also form in the kidneys and cause kidney stones.

There is no cure for gout, but it can and should be controlled in order to avoid pain and permanent damage to afflicted areas. People prone to gout are usually advised to limit their intake of foods and beverages that are high in purines, such as anchovies, beer, gravies, kidneys, liver, sardines and wines. In addition, they can take certain drugs to reduce their uric acid levels and control gout symptoms.

However, these drugs can produce unpleasant side effects.[126-131]

Fortunately, *Rhododendron caucasicum* can regulate uric acid levels and relieve gout symptoms without the unpleasant side effects. Drs. Ramazanov and del Mar Bernal Suarez reported on this use for the plant in their book. They noted that *Rhododendron caucasicum* has been used to treat gout for many centuries, and then they went on to outline the clinical studies that prove the rhododendron extract's effectiveness at treating. In one clinical study performed by professor D. M. Rossiisskiy, M.D., of the Russian Medical Academy on 170 volunteers who had severe attacks of gout, rhododendron extract increased the discharge of uric acid through urination. In just a few hours, after only five or six doses of the extract, the pain and disagreeable symptoms associated with gout were relieved.[2,6,125,129,132] In another clinical study, Soviet doctors A. D. Samartzev, I. V. Aushev, and F. R. Israelov at Dagestan State Hospital gave 150 milligrams of rhododendron extract to 320 volunteers who were suffering from severe attacks of gout. The initial test dose increased the amount of uric acid elimination by between 35 percent and 60 percent. Furthermore, continued treatment helped prevent further gout suffering.[125,129,133]

In addition to increasing uric acid discharge, rhododendron extract may also improve the functioning of the gout sufferers' livers. To understand how, we must first explain that uric acid is produced by the liver. Therefore, the liver must function properly to produce and process uric acid as it should. However, because the liver is the body's primary purification and detoxification organ, it is constantly subjected to damage by the toxins and free radicals that enter it. Over time, accumulated toxic waste and free radical damage can cause the liver to malfunction. Scientists believe this malfunctioning may contribute to the up to 30 percent of gout episodes that are caused by uric acid overproduction.[134,135]

For many years, vitamin E has been deemed the best protector and detoxifying nutrient for the liver. However, recent research now shows that the flavonoid taxifolin, a key constituent of *Rhododendron caucasicum*, is a far better defender and detoxifier of the liver than even vitamin E.[2,136,137]

GLAUCOMA

Glaucoma has been defined as "vision growing gray,"[138] but the term actually represents a number of disorders that, in most cases, are characterized by increased eye pressure. This increased pressure damages the eye and leads to blindness. Now, an estimated 67 million people worldwide, including 3 million Americans, suffer from glaucoma. Every year, more than 100,000 Americans develop the disorder, and every day without treatment takes them closer to blindness. Today, glaucoma is the third leading cause of blindness worldwide, and an estimated 120,000 Americans are now blind as a result of the disease.[139,140,141]

What specifically causes glaucoma? The disorder is related to the drainage of eye fluids. One such fluid, aqueous humor, constantly circulates through the eye, delivering nutrients and oxygen to the lens and cornea, collecting waste, and then draining into the bloodstream. This constant circulation ensures that the pressure the fluid creates within the eye remains constant as well. However, decreases in the quantity and quality of nutrients available to the eye's drainage system can cause the system to lose its permeability and elasticity and become blocked. When eye fluid ceases to drain off, pressure builds in the eye. This pressure compresses the cells of the retina and the one million cells of the optic nerve. Over time, these cells are damaged and die, and vision is lost. But because the loss of vision is painless and gradual, victims usually don't recognize the problem until it has progressed to an advanced stage.[138,142,143]

For many centuries, *Rhododendron caucasicum* has been used in Georgian folk medicine to treat various age-related and vision-degenerative disorders, including glaucoma, and for decades scientists have wondered why *Rhododendron caucasicum* is so effective at treating elevated inner eye pressure. Now, new research shows that *Rhododendron caucasicum's* recently identified taxifolins might be responsible.[2]

In one study, taxifolins were given to patients who had glaucoma, sclerotic macular dystrophia (progressive hardening of the retinal tissue due to inadequate nutrition), and diabetic and hypertension angioretinopathia (retinal destruction). These patients were given 20 milligrams of taxifolins four times a day for thirty days. At the end of the trial period, researchers noted that all the patients exhibited improvements in the sharpness of their vision and improvements in the sensibility and conduction of their optic nerves. In addition, the patients' fields of vision increased by between ten and fifteen feet.[2]

Scientists at the Russian Medicinal Academy of Science's Eye Microsurgery Institute also studied taxifolins treatment for glaucoma patients. Their clinical trials revealed that taxifolins prevented additional damage to the eye's cellular membranes and to the permeability of the eye's drainage system. Thus, taxifolins, as found in *Rhododendron caucasicum*, inhibited the eye tissue damage caused by poor access to nutrients.[2]

But taxifolins have also been shown to have other positive effects on the eyes and to treat other visual disorders. For example, sorbitol is a sweet-tasting sugar alcohol that often is used as a substitute for sugar. Sorbitol also is formed from glucose in the body. High levels of glucose or sorbital in the bloodsteam results in a build up of sorbitol in the cells, which is associated with cellular dysfunction, tissue damage, nerve dysfunction, cataracts, and vascular damage of the retina.[144-147] But Japanese scientists have demonstrated that taxifolins help prevent the conversion of glucose to sorbitol. Taxifolins have also been shown to keep sorbitol from accumulating in red blood cells.[148] And in another study, this one performed on rats whose eye lenses had been incubated with a high concentration of glucose, taxifolins maintained the lenses' clarity. This is important because it further indicates that taxifolins may be effective at preventing the eye damage that comes from hyperglycemia.[149,150] All in all, these discoveries clearly indicate that consuming plants or herbs that contain high amounts of taxifolins (and *Rhododendron caucasicum* is one such plant) might help promote good vision.

BACTERIAL INFECTIONS

Most species of bacteria are not harmful and, in fact, are essential to life on earth. However, several species of bacteria have been responsible for decimating entire civilizations. As recently as the late 1800s, more than a quarter of all children in the United States died of bacterial infections before reaching puberty.[151,152,153]

Today that percentage has been substantially reduced in developed nations, but bacterial infections still pose a significant threat to our health. Each year, millions of Americans suffer from bouts of strep throat, 73,000 cases of *E. coli* (Escherichia coli) infections appear, and staph and other pathogenic infections make hospitals dangerous places in which to be sick.[154-157] During 1995, in New York City alone,

Table 5. Activity of Rhododendron Extract against Harmful Bacteria

Substance	Amount added to bacteria colony	24 hour test	Staphylococcus aureus	Bacillus anthracoldes	Escherichia coli
Rhododendron Caucasicum extract	10 mg.	Number of bacteria colonies at beginning of test=	12,000	2,900	2,120
Bacteria colonies surviving at end of 24 hour test=			0	12	25

Substance	Amount added to bacteria colony	24 hour test	Bacillus disenteriae	Bacillus proteus	Streptococcus haemolyticus
Rhododendron caucasicum extract	10 mg.	Number of bacteria colonies at beginning of test=	1,900	9,000	1,100
Bacteria colonies surviving at end of 24 hour test=			0	0	0

Source: Zakir Ramazanov, Ph.D. 1997. 125,132

13,500 hospital patients became infected with *Staphylococcus aureus*, which cost the city more than $430 million. More alarming, the death rate of those patients infected with staph was more than double the death rate of uninfected patients.[154] And this isn't just a New York problem. The rate at which patients acquired infections in American hospitals rose 36 percent between 1975 and 1995. Of the 36 million people admitted to U.S. hospitals during 1995, 1.8 million were infected with bacteria while in the hospital, and these infections contributed to more than 88,000 patient deaths.[158] During the year 2000, "about 103,000 patient deaths were linked to hospital-acquired infections, making these infections the fourth leading cause of death in the United States," according to the *Chicago Tribune*.[159]

Most alarming is the fact that many strains of pathogenic bacteria are becoming progressively resistant to drug treatments.[158,160,161,162] During the spring of 2003, Neil Fishman, M.D., director of the Department of Healthcare Epidemiology and Infection Control at the University of Pennsylvania Medical Center estimated that antibiotic-resistant bacteria now cause 19,000 deaths in the United States every year.[163] And the problem will likely get worse, especially since not one of the eighty-nine F.D.A.-approved drugs of 2002 was an antibiotic and only five of the more than four hundred drugs currently in development are antibiotics.[163]

But there is good news to report, too, and it comes from *Rhododendron caucasicum*, which has been used for hundreds of years in Georgian folk medicine to prevent and treat bacterial infections. One of the plant's rather unique adaptogenic qualities is that it allows probiotics, or good bacteria (such as those that exist in yogurt and in our intestines), to survive and thrive, while at the same time, it actively fights many pathogenic bacteria.[20,125,132] In fact, table 5 shows rhododendron extract's activity against pathogenic bacteria in tests performed in vitro.

The results shown in table 5, and the fact that for centuries Georgians have used the plant for exactly this purpose, indicate that *Rhododendron caucasicum* may provide an effective first line of defense against harmful bacteria.[20]

Choosing a Rhododendron Extract

At this point, *Rhododendron caucasicum*'s potential health benefits are clear. However, it is important to note that not every rhododendron extract will provide such benefits. In fact, some rhododendron species may be hazardous if ingested. For that reason, please note that Georgian-grown *Rhododendron caucasicum* spring leaves extract is safe and possesses the unique properties described herein.

And what makes this extract better than other natural extracts that might also improve human health? There are several superior properties. For one thing, *Rhododendron caucasicum* spring leaves extract is biologically friendly.[2] It won't interfere with other important metabolic functions and processes, such as the absorption and metabolism of essential nutrients, vitamins, and minerals. Beyond that, the extract is also bioavailable, and it is made without the use of toxic organic solvents.

BIOAVAILABILITY

In order for substances to be effective as antioxidants in internal body organs and tissues, they must be bioavailable—able to be absorbed and ready for physiological use after administration. Most people assume that a substance is

Table 6. Antioxidant Values

Raw Material	Phenolic Content	Plasma serum Antioxidant value
Rhododendron spring leaves extract (low in OPC's)	50%	62%
Rhododendron summer-fall leaves extract (high in OPC's)	70%	5%
Placebo control group	0%	0%

Source: Zakir Ramazanov, Ph.D. 2000.[2,166]

bioavailable if it's able to cross the intestinal membrane. But true bioavailability is actually determined by the percentage of a substance that has crossed the intestinal membrane, traveled to the liver, and reentered circulating blood intact after passage through the liver.

Nutritional companies often advertise the bioavailability and antioxidant activity of their products based upon simple "test tube" studies. Georgian scientists, though, realize that bioavailability of an antioxidant must be determined by the antioxidant's activity in blood serum.

Nutritional companies also often infer that the antioxidant activity of a product is equivalent to the phenolic content of a product. But as previously stated, high phenolic content, though indicative of high antioxidant activity, is not necessarily analogous to high antioxidant activity. Only certain special phenolics are antioxidants, while many other phenolics produce no antioxidant activity whatsoever. Furthermore, as also mentioned, the phenolic composition of plants varies according to species, growing conditions, etc., and the bioavailability and antioxidant values of different antioxidant phenolics vary as well. The variances even within a single species of plant can be quite surprising.[2,8,164,165,166] In the case of *Rhododendron caucasicum*, for instance, the following variation in phenolic content is observed:

Rhododendron caucasicum spring leaves, harvested during March, are high in hydroxycinnamic, chlorogenic, and gallic acid derivatives, and taxifolins. They lack oligomeric proanthocyanidins (OPCs), the phenolics in grape seed and pine bark extracts. The total phenolic content of *Rhododendron caucasicum* spring leaves extract is 50 percent.

Rhododendron caucasicum summer-fall leaves, harvested during late September, consist of 30 percent to 35 percent OPCs. These leaves are low in simple phenolic acids and are virtually devoid of taxifolins. However, the total phenolic content of *Rhododendron caucasicum* summer-fall leaves extract is 70 percent.[2]

Most people would assume that the extract with the higher total phenolic content (70 percent versus 50 percent) and the one that consists of 30 percent to 35 percent OPCs would display the highest antioxidant activity and be the most bioavailable. But that is not the case, as research has proved.

Drs. Ramazanov and del Mar Bernal Suarez reported on this research in their book. They wrote: "In a Soviet study, 200 milligrams of rhododendron extract obtained from both spring and summer-fall leaves were given to two separate groups of 107 volunteers. Blood serum samples were collected to determine the antioxidant status of plasma, measured by the total radical-trapping antioxidant parameter. A control group received 200 milliliters of water."[2,166]

As shown in table 6, the extract with the higher phenolic content, which also had the highest OPC content, had a plasma serum antioxidant value of 5 percent—which was hardly higher than the control group, which received only water. The rhododendron spring leaves extract, which lacked OPCs but contained high amounts of hydroxycinnamic, chlorogenic, and gallic acid derivatives and taxifolins, showed an extremely high plasma serum antioxidant value of 62 percent.

According to the researchers, the difference in the antioxidant values was due to the fact that "OPCs are not as effectively absorbed from our diets, as they form insoluble complexes with macromolecules such as proteins and carbohydrates. OPCs are less permeable to membranes, both because of their size and [because of their] relative polarity."[166,167,168] In other words, OPCs aren't as bioavailable as the special phenolics—relatively small-sized molecules of antioxidant flavonoids and phenolic acids—found in rhododendron spring leaves extract. These highly active antioxidants are more bioavailable for humans than large molecules of OPCs.[166]

EXTRACTION

As explained in the Introduction, almost all antioxidant compounds sold today are extracted with toxic organic solvents. Perfect examples are grape seed and pine bark extracts, sold under several different names, which became well-known during the early 1990s as sources of proanthocyanadins (the "PC" in OPCs).[169]

Producing grape seed and pine bark extracts almost always involves the use of toxic organic solvents.[2,132,170,171,172] These solvents cannot be completely removed from the substances

Table 7. Chemical Analysis: Toxic Organic Solvent Residue PPM

Extract	Chloroform	Butanol	Ethylacetate
Rhododendron caucasicum extract	0	0	0
Grape Seed extract	50	40	21
Pine Bark extract	50	27	13

Gas chromatographic analysis to determine the parts per million (PPM) of organic solvents found in substances/products following processing.

Source: Zakir Ramazanov, Ph.D., 1997.[125,132]

after the extraction process is complete, so the toxic residue remains in the end products and is consumed day after day by the public. The irony is that grape seed extract and pine bark extracts are purchased, in part, because of their free radical neutralizing properties. However, the toxic organic solvent residues that those same products almost always contain produce free radicals. Therefore, some of these extracts' free radical neutralizing activity is spent cleaning up the very free radicals they introduce.[8,20,125,132]

Rhododendron caucasicum spring leaves extract contains far more effective free radical neutralizers and not even a trace of toxic organic solvents—because no toxic organic solvents are used in its extraction or processing. The antioxidants in *Rhododendron caucasicum* extract are extracted using only water and a high-pressure filtration technique.[166] If a solvent other than water must be used in an extraction process, it should be a nontoxic solvent, such as ethyl alcohol, the type of alcohol in wine.

Based on the aforementioned, and for reasons of both

effectiveness and value, consumers should be sure that a rhododendron extract product meets the following specifications:

- The product is made from the rhododendron species *Rhododendron caucasicum*.
- The plants used in the product were grown at high altitudes of the Caucasian Mountains in Georgia.
- The plants' leaves were harvested in the spring, when they were young.
- The plants were grown in the wild without the use of herbicides or pesticides.
- The product does not contain toxic solvents; instead, water and high-pressure filtration were used for extraction.
- The product meets the standard of containing at least 40 percent phenolics, of which at least 5 percent are taxifolins.

Ancient Wisdom, Modern Science

Long-living Georgians have demonstrated *Rhododendron caucasicum*'s safety and health-protecting properties by using this plant for some 2,000 years. In addition, the plant has been a staple of Georgian folk medicine for more than 1,500 years. But consumers don't have to rely solely on folk medicine to realize *Rhododendron caucasicum*'s benefits. As has been shown, over the last fifty years, the plant's safety and its medicinal properties have been demonstrated and confirmed in modern biochemical, toxicological, pharmacological, and clinical studies performed at leading scientific research centers. Clearly, then, this plant can make a difference in people's health and very likely extend their lives.

As mentioned at the beginning of the chapter,

Rhododendron caucasicum is one of the four most important health-promoting, antiaging plants that traditional Georgians used for centuries. Next, we'll explore each of the other three plants—Caucasian blueberry leaves, Georgian pomegranate, and *Rhodiola rosea*. Each provides remarkable protection for the health of the entire body.

CHAPTER 4

Caucasian Blueberry Leaves

The Caucasian blueberry plant, *Vaccinium arctostaphylos L*, is a large, berry-producing bush that grows wild at altitudes of 3,000 feet to 5,000 feet in the Caucasus Mountains.[1,2] It is, in fact, indigenous to the these mountains, as is another species of blueberry, *Vaccinium myrtillus L*. As previously described, the chemical composition of any plant species is largely the result of environment, so not surprisingly, by growing in the same area, these two species have become nearly identical to one another in chemical composition. Therefore, the two species are now collectively known by many nonscientists as Caucasian blueberry, but only when their growth occurred on the Caucasian Mountains of Georgia.[3]

Georgians are believed to have been consuming delicious teas made from the leaves of the Caucasian blueberry plant since well before the reach of recorded history. In addition, teas made with Caucasian blueberry leaves have been used in Georgian folk medicine for at least 600 years.[3]

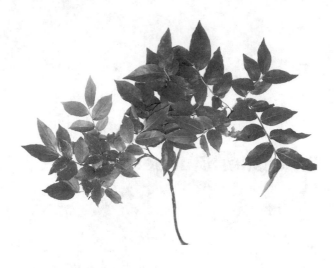

Caucasian blueberry spring leaves

As Professor Musa Abidoff, M.D., of the Moscow Center for Modern Medicine, has noted, the primary use of Caucasian blueberry leaves in Georgian folk medicine has been in the prevention and treatment of diabetes and other sugar imbalances.[1,2,3] In fact, Abidoff says the blueberry leaves have a "legendary reputation as an aid to diabetics" and that teas made with these leaves are commonly referred to as "antidiabetes teas."[1] Dr. Zakir Ramazanov also notes that in Eurasia Caucasian blueberry leaves tea is widely known as the "Georgian diabetes remedy."[3] Additionally, in eastern Europe, including areas of Russia, a standardized Caucasian blueberry leaves extract tea, Diabetic Chai Cherniki, is effectively used to treat diabetes, high cholesterol, and digestive problems, including gastric colitis.[1,4,5] Traditional Caucasian blueberry leaves teas have also been used to sooth sore throats and treat diarrhea and urinary tract infections.[2,6]

Interestingly, today, Caucasian blueberry leaves extract is beginning to be used by Westerners to minimize "sugar crashes" and after-meal tiredness and crankiness—and to maintain healthy glucose levels.

Chemical Makeup of Caucasian Blueberry Leaves

Caucasian blueberry leaves' phytochemical composition has been studied at the Georgian Academy of Sciences for decades. These investigations have shown that the leaves contain large amounts of two well-researched and widely sought plant chemicals, namely chlorogenic acid and hydroxycinnamic acid.[1-5] Since the mid-1960s, these powerful phenolic antioxidants have been described in more than 1,800 pharmacological and clinical studies published in scientific journals worldwide.[7]

Additional scientific studies have shown that the volume of chlorogenic acid and hydroxycinnamic acid in the leaves depends upon the plant's growth period. For example, research completed during 1971 and 1972 by Georgian plant physiologist V. V. Mshavanadze, Ph.D., and her colleagues at the Georgian Academy of Sciences revealed that the concentration of chlorogenic and hydroxycinnamic acids can be as high as 28 percent in young Caucasian blueberry leaves. However, the concentration drops to between 1 and 3 percent in mature summer leaves.[4,8] These findings have been repeatedly substantiated by subsequent research over the last thirty years.[9]

In light of the findings, Caucasian blueberry leaves are now harvested in early spring to ensure that they have the highest possible concentrations of chlorogenic and hydroxycinnamic acids. High concentrations of these phenolics guarantee that the plant extract will produce optimal medicinal effects.[1,4,5]

Interestingly, when used in Georgian folk medicine, the leaves were also harvested in the spring.[3]

True Caucasian blueberry leaves extract is standardized to contain a minimum of 20 percent chlorogenic and hydroxycinnamic acids, although the actual concentration of these two important nutrients is usually higher than the minimums listed on the labels.[9] The leaves also contain a host of other important nutrients.[6,10] One or more of these additional nutrients may act synergistically with chlorogenic and hydroxycinnamic acids to help produce or enhance Caucasian blueberry leaves' famed antidiabetes effect.[3]

Next, we'll explore that effect in more detail by examining what causes diabetes and how Caucasian blueberry leaves might help prevent and treat the disease.

Diabetes

The term "diabetes" refers to a group of complex chronic diseases that affect an estimated 15.7 million to 20.8 million Americans.[11,12] The disease is related to the way in which sugar, or glucose, is processed in our bodies.

Glucose is the basic fuel our cells use to create energy. The hormone insulin, which is created by the pancreas, transports glucose from our blood into our cells. Sometimes, though, the pancreas doesn't produce enough insulin, or cells become less sensitive to insulin. When this happens, the cells don't absorb the glucose, which instead remains in the blood, building to dangerous levels. A chronic abundance of glucose damages the body's blood vessels, which leads to a functional breakdown of organs. This kind of chronic glucose abundance, caused by insulin imbalance or loss of insulin sensitivity, is called diabetes.[13,14]

Type 1 diabetes, previously called insulin-dependent diabetes or juvenile-onset diabetes, develops when the body's
immune system destroys pancreatic beta cells—the cells that
make insulin. This form of diabetes usually strikes children
and young adults, who need several insulin injections a day
(or an insulin pump) to survive. Type 1 diabetes accounts for
5 percent to 10 percent of all diagnosed cases of diabetes, and
autoimmune disorders, genetic predisposition, and environmental factors are usually involved in its development.[13,15]

When diabetes develops later in life, it's usually because
cells have become less sensitive to insulin—a problem that is
often aggravated by glucose overproduction in the liver. As
the need for insulin rises, the pancreas gradually wears down
and loses its ability to produce insulin. This condition is called
Type 2 or adult-onset diabetes.[13]

Both forms of diabetes bring serious, deleterious health
consequences. For instance, if left untreated, diabetes can
cause retinal degeneration and blindness, lead to kidney and
nerve damage, and contribute to atherosclerosis. In extreme
cases, it can even result in amputation and death.

The statistics showing the prevalence of such events are
ominous. Between twelve thousand and twenty-four thousand Americans lose their sight each year because of diabetes.
In addition, between 27,900 and 42,800 diabetics suffer kidney failure each year. Diabetics are also two to four times
more likely to suffer from heart disease, two to four times
more likely to have a stroke, and three times more likely to
die of complications from flu or pneumonia than nondiabet-
ics. And between 56,000 and 82,000 lower limb amputations
are performed on diabetics each year.[16,17]

Also alarming is the fact that the number of diabetics has
increased in recent decades. Between 1958 and 1997, while
the U.S. population increased by 46 percent, the number of

Americans diagnosed with diabetes increased by a staggering 643 percent.[18,19] During 1997, diabetes was the eighth most frequently diagnosed adverse health condition. Only three years later, by the end of the year 2000, diabetes had become the third most frequently diagnosed adverse health condition.[20] During 2001, about 798,000 Americans were newly diagnosed with diabetes, and the disease was the sixth leading cause of death in the United States.[11,16] However, during November of 2003, the National Institute of Diabetes and Digestive and Kidney Diseases reported that 1.3 million American adults had been newly diagnosed with diabetes during 2002.[21,22] All told, the cost of health care and lost productivity due to diabetes totaled about $132 billion in 2003.[22]

Not only is the number of Americans afflicted with Type 2 diabetes increasing at an alarming rate, but the disease is also striking at younger ages. In the past, Type 2 diabetes rarely struck before middle age (forty years of age or older); now, it is sneaking up on young adults and children, frequently causing permanent damage even before it is diagnosed.[16,23] The most recent statistics from the Centers for Disease Control and Prevention show that between 1990 and 1998, the number of 30- to 39-year-old Americans with Type 2 diabetes increased by 76 percent. And American children as young as four years old are now being diagnosed with Type 2 diabetes.[24]

SUGAR CONSUMPTION AND DIABETES

Some scientists still disagree about whether excessive sugar consumption contributes to the onset of chronic hypoglycemia and nondiabetic hyperglycemia, or to Type 2 diabetes itself. However, statistics show a correlation between increases in sugar consumption and increases in the number of people with diabetes. This correlation seems to indicate at least some kind of cause-and-effect relationship between sugar consumption and the disease.

Increases in sugar consumption. In the past 150 years, American sugar consumption has grown considerably. In 1840, for instance, each American consumed, on average, about four teaspoons of sweeteners per day, or about thirteen pounds of sugar per year.[25] But over time, sugar consumption increased so much that by 1999 each American consumed an average twenty teaspoons of sugar per day, or sixty-four pounds of sugar per year. That's an 800 percent increase in per capita sugar consumption since 1840, and a 30 percent increase since 1983. And the age-specific statistics are even worse. For example, by 1999, the average American teenage boy consumed thirty-four teaspoons of sugar per day, or about 109 pounds of sugar per year.[26]

Notably, the statistics don't include the massive amounts of carbohydrates the average American consumes each year from breads, grains, cereals, beans, french fries, milk, beer, and other foods. Almost 90 percent of the carbohydrates we consume from these sources enter the blood as glucose as well.[27]

Increases in diabetes. As sugar (and carbohydrate) consumption has increased, the number of people diagnosed with diabetes has also gone up. Some of the early statistics on the number of diabetes cases were gathered in 1959. Notably, during the following seven years, or from 1959 to 1966, the number of Americans with diabetes increased by 67 percent, and large percentage gains continued through the 1960s, 1970s, and 1980s.[15] More recently, between 1990 and 1998, the number of Americans with diabetes increased by 33 percent. At the end of that period, in 1998, the disease affected 6.5 percent of the U.S. population (up from 4.9 percent in

1990).[16] By 2000, the number of diabetic Americans had risen to 7.3 percent of the population. Increases were observed in people of both sexes and among all ages, ethnic groups, and educational levels.[28]

In a January 2002 statement published in the journal *Diabetes Care*, the American Diabetes Association projected that the prevalence of diabetes will rise to 9 percent of the adult population before the year 2026.[29] As startling as that rather near-term estimate is, the implications of long-term projections are even more horrifying. One such projection was given in June 2003 by Venkat Narayan, M.D., M.P.H., an epidemiologist specializing in diabetes research for the Centers for Disease Control and Prevention. Dr. Narayan announced that, based on new insight into current trends, 33 percent of children born during the year 2000 will likely develop diabetes by the year 2050—and he added that this estimate was "probably quite conservative."[30]

If the Centers for Disease Control and Prevention's projections hold true—and all indications are that they will—one out of every three adult Americans will suffer from the severely debilitating and ultimately deadly effects of diabetes within a mere blink of time. And these projections do not include the tens of millions of additional Americans who may be suffering from hypoglycemia or nondiabetic hyperglycemia.[17,31] The damage diabetes will soon do to people's lives, our society, and the U.S. economy, not to mention the strain it will create on the American health care system, could be overwhelming. As Dr. Kevin McKinney, director of the Adult Clinical Endocrinological Unit at the University of Texas Medical Center in Galveston, Texas, noted in commenting on the Centers for Disease Control's findings, "There is no way the medical community can keep up with that."[30]

Sugar and glucose levels. Clearly, then, the number of diabetics in the United States has increased as Americans' sugar consumption has increased. But how are the two related?

As most everyone knows, sugar increases glucose levels. Consuming it therefore results in at least gradual harm to the body, even for people who currently feel fine. Eating sugar-laden foods and drinks, not to mention excessive amounts of carbohydrates, forces the pancreas to constantly work overtime to produce enough insulin to process the glucose. And as noted previously, when insulin levels stay high for a prolonged period of time, the body's tissues become less sensitive to it, or even resistant to it, which requires the pancreas to produce even more insulin. As the need for insulin rises, the pancreas gradually wears down and loses its ability to produce insulin. This results in chronic high blood glucose levels, which age us by damaging the body's blood vessels and which thereby degenerate body organs and systems.[32,33] In other words, chronic high blood glucose levels result in diabetes.

If sugar raises glucose levels and high glucose levels cause diabetes, it therefore seems reasonable to say that excess sugar consumption can cause diabetes. In fact, many scientists now believe just that. They also believe that by raising blood glucose levels, sugar may promote the development of or increase the severity of heart disease, depression, attention deficit disorder, kidney disease, colon cancer, gallstones, obesity, and ulcers. This is because of sugar's chemical activity and because of the nutrition it replaces.[34,35,36]

Illness and glucose levels. While sugar's role in the development of diabetes is extremely important, it is also important to note that illness itself can raise glucose levels, even in people who previously haven't suffered from diabetes or nondiabetic hyperglycemia. Critically ill patients, especially, are often subject to significant increases in glucose levels, and these increases can have serious consequences.[37] Conversely, when critically ill patients' blood glucose levels are kept in check, their risk of serious complications is dramatically reduced. This phenomenon was shown in a randomized, controlled study conducted at Catholic University in Leuven, Belgium. Researchers monitored and controlled the blood glucose levels of 1,548 intensive care patients. Approximately half the patients were assigned to receive blood-glucose-lowering therapy in order to keep their blood glucose at normal levels— between 80 and 110 milligrams per deciliter. The rest of the intensive care patients received blood-glucose-lowering therapy only if their blood glucose levels exceeded 215 milligrams per deciliter, and then only to lower glucose levels to, and maintain them at, between 180 and 200 milligrams per deciliter. The result? The patients whose blood glucose levels were maintained at normal amounts were 42 percent less likely to die. They also had 46 percent fewer bloodstream infections, 41 percent fewer acute kidney failures requiring dialysis or hemofiltration, 50 percent fewer red blood cell transfusions, and 44 percent fewer diseases of the nervous system.[37]

The fact is, for all people—sick and well alike—reducing blood glucose levels to normal amounts results in less glucose-induced damage to blood vessels, lower insulin requirements, a slowing of the onset of insulin insensitivity, less wear on the pancreas, and better overall health. In the face of such results, it is clear that keeping one's blood glucose levels in check should be a priority for everyone.

PREVENTING AND COMBATING DIABETES

To maintain healthy glucose levels, all Americans should exercise, dramatically reduce their sugar consumption, eat at least three nutritious meals per day, and never allow themselves to be hungry. In other words, for many people, a possible way to slow the onset of diabetes, hypoglycemia, and non-diabetic hyperglycemia may be to eat and exercise as though they are already diabetic—or, in other words, to eat and exercise as long-living traditional Georgians have for centuries.

American anthropologist Sula Benet, whose work has been noted in previous chapters, experienced the effects of choosing such a lifestyle. She spent a great deal of time with long-living Caucasians, exercising and eating as they did. Of her time in the Caucasus, she wrote: "Sugar was totally absent from my diet, with only an occasional bit of honey. Without any conscious effort, I lost ten pounds during the first three weeks and felt physically strong and energetic." In addition, when she returned to the United States, she wrote: "The physical benefits . . . of unaccustomed physical exertion . . . were quite apparent on my return, when I found that stairways that I might usually avoid were easy to climb."[38]

For those whose blood glucose levels are already high, Dr. Zakir Ramazanov explains the medical approach that is typically used to keep glucose levels in check. He says, "The prime objective in the treatment of diabetes is to lower abnormally high levels of blood glucose to normal levels, and then to stabilize the blood glucose at those normal levels. Three therapeutic strategies are generally used to achieve this:

1. Reduce glucose absorption from the diet.
2. Reduce glucose synthesis in the liver.
3. Accelerate glucose metabolism."[10]

Ideally, the most effective strategy in fighting diabetes would be to achieve all three of these objectives at the same time. Fortunately, traditional Georgians found a way to do just that.

In addition to being physically active and eating healthy foods, traditional Georgians used a unique substance to help control their glucose levels. That substance was Caucasian blueberry leaves. These leaves served as a treatment for diabetes, and many believe it can help prevent hypoglycemia, hyperglycemia, and Type 2 diabetes as well. This is because Caucasian blueberry leaves can help the body achieve all three of Dr. Ramazanov's therapeutic strategies.

What makes Caucasian blueberry leaves so effective against diabetes? The answer lies in the plant's high concentrations of two phenolic antioxidants: chlorogenic acid and hydroxycinnamic acid.

Help from chlorogenic and hydroxycinnamic acids. New studies suggest that chlorogenic and hydroxycinnamic acids help reduce dietary glucose absorption, help reduce glucose synthesis in the liver, and speed up glucose metabolism.[10]

In a study on glucose absorption, researchers at Rutgers University compared chlorogenic acid and hydroxycinnamic acid with other phenolics. Specifically, the scientists monitored these phenolics' abilities to reduce glucose absorption in the small intestine. In the end, chlorogenic acid reduced glucose absorption up to 80 percent, and hydroxycinnamic acid reduced absorption to between 30 percent and 40 percent. The other phenolics had no effect on glucose absorption.[39]

Research has also shown that chlorogenic acid helps reduce glucose synthesis.[10] This is because of the way in which the phenolic interacts with a key glucose-regulating enzyme. The enzyme glucose-6-phosphatase (G6P) is responsible for glucose formation in our bodies, and scientists recently discovered that chlorogenic acid could inhibit this key enzyme's activity in the liver. This is excellent news, because inhibiting G6P activity in the liver means this organ produces less glucose. Therefore, as reported in the *Archives of Biochemistry and Biophysics* and in *The Journal of Medical Chemistry*, chlorogenic acid can be used to reduce the abnormally high liver glucose output often found in non-insulin-dependent diabetics.[40,41] Pharmaceutical companies have already created several synthetic versions of chlorogenic acid for this purpose. These potent compounds have also been shown to inhibit G6P activity in human liver microsomes.[42] In addition, German research has revealed that chlorogenic acid-based compounds inhibited glucose synthesis in isolated rat liver tissue.[43]

Another study, this one conducted in Taiwan, showed hydroxycinnamic acid's effect on glucose metabolism. As reported in the German journal *Naunyn-Schmiedebergs Archives of Pharmacology*, hydroxycinnamic acid accelerated glucose metabolism,[44] and as Dr. Ramazanov points out, this metabolic acceleration can reduce the total glucose concentration circulating in blood.[3]

Results of additional Taiwanese studies on diabetic rats provide further evidence that hydroxycinnamic acid might reduce blood glucose levels.[45] And German researchers recently provided evidence that chlorogenic acid derivatives can reduce blood glucose levels in fasting rats, which confirms the blood-glucose-lowering properties of chlorogenic acid.[46] Clearly, then, based on these scientific studies, chlorogenic and hydroxycinnamic acids can play an important role in preventing and treating diabetes, although, as Dr. Ramazanov notes, their effectiveness may depend on whether the compounds are taken simultaneously and whether they are consumed in sufficient amounts.[3,10]

Many North American scientists will probably be surprised to learn that chlorogenic and hydroxycinnamic acids—which have elicited so much recent excitement—were discovered decades ago in Caucasian blueberry leaves, the centuries-old Georgian folk medicine diabetes remedy. Even so, by testing the concentrations of these phenolics in Caucasian blueberry leaves and discovering that those concentrations are extremely high, we realize today that Caucasian blueberry spring leaves are the world's most abundant source of these highly important phytochemicals.[3] They are what make Caucasian blueberry leaves so effective against diabetes.

Research on Caucasian blueberry leaves extract. In addition to the scientific studies on Caucasian blueberry leaves' two most powerful antioxidant phenolics, tests have also measured the effectiveness of an extract made from the leaves. These studies on both animals and humans have further demonstrated the extract's ability to lower glucose levels and ultimately fight diabetes.

In one such study on rats, Italian researchers at the University of Milan studied the therapeutic action of blueberry leaves extract by administering it to streptozotocin-diabetic rats for four days. Glucose levels were consistently found to drop by about 26 percent at two different stages of diabetes. Unexpectedly, triglyceride levels also decreased by 39 percent following treatment.[47] These results indicate that blueberry leaves' active constituents may prove useful in treating both diabetes and high triglycerides. And as suspected, the findings also suggest that the active constituents of blueberry leaves extract might be involved in regulating blood glucose synthesis.[47]

Caucasian blueberry leaves extract has also been tested on healthy human volunteers. For example, Russian scientist

Musa T. Abidoff, M.D., evaluated the glucose-lowering properties of blueberry leaves extract in a double blind, placebo-
controlled study at the Moscow Center for Modern
Medicine.[2] Seventy-five healthy volunteers between the ages
of 37 and 64 years were invited to participate in the five-
week trial. Sixty days before beginning the drug phase of this
trial, the volunteers went through a period of diet counseling and surveillance. Their diets were standardized so that 55
percent to 60 percent of their calories came from carbohydrates, and at three-week intervals throughout the study, the
volunteers' fasting plasma glucose values were evaluated,
their food records were analyzed, and their symptoms were
recorded. Then, after the initial dietary phase, subjects were
also randomly assigned to receive either 150 milligrams of
blueberry leaves extract or a placebo three times a day
(taken with water before meals). In the end, volunteers in
the placebo group saw their average blood glucose level
increase to 142 milligrams per deciliter from 102 milligrams
per deciliter. In contrast, volunteers taking blueberry leaves
extract saw their average glucose level increase to only 121

Table 8. Caucasian Blueberry Leaves: Glucose Study 1

	Placebo Group
Before Meal Glucose Level	102
After Meal Glucose Level	142

	Blueberry Leaves Extract Group
Before Meal Glucose Level	109
After Meal Glucose Level	121

Source: Musa T. Abidoff, M.D., 1999.[2]

Table 9. Caucasian Blueberry Leaves: Glucose Study 2

Placebo Group

Before Meal Glucose Level	84
After Meal Glucose Level	120

Blueberry Leaves Extract Group

Before Meal Glucose Level	84
After Meal Glucose Level	105

Source: Musa T. Abidoff, M.D., 1999.[1]

Table 10. Caucasian Blueberry Leaves: Glucose Study 3

Beginning of Study: Prior to Blueberry Leaves Applications Mean Plasma Glucose Level

169

End of Study: After Blueberry Leaves Applications Mean Plasma Glucose Level

136

Source: Musa T. Abidoff, M.D., 1999.[2]

milligrams per deciliter from 109 milligrams per deciliter. This difference indicates that the blueberry leaves extract possessed physiologically significant glucose-lowering properties.

Dr. Abidoff also conducted a second double-blind, placebo-controlled clinical trial using the extract. In this second trial, fifty-two healthy volunteers between the ages of twenty-five and seventy-two were selected to receive 300 milligrams of Caucasian blueberry leaves extract three times per day (taken with water just before meals). Volunteers in the placebo group saw their after-meal glucose levels increase to an average 120 milligrams per deciliter from 85 milligrams per deciliter, while those volunteers taking Caucasian blueberry leaves extract saw their after-meal glucose levels increase to an average of only 105 milligrams per deciliter from 84 milligrams per deciliter.[1] According to Dr. Abidoff, the Caucasian blueberry leaves extract's glucose-lowering effect was due to its chlorogenic acid. And as other scientists had also discovered, Dr. Abidoff found that chlorogenic acid appeared to inhibit the activity of the G6P enzyme in glucose production.[1]

Finally, in a third clinical trial, Dr. Abidoff observed the effects of Caucasian blueberry leaves extract on the plasma glucose levels of Type 2 diabetics.[2] Twenty-nine patients, average age fifty years old and all with Type 2 diabetes, were selected to participate in this double-blind, placebo-controlled, sixty-day trial. Two months before beginning the drug phase of the clinical study, the patients went through a period of diet counseling and surveillance wherein their dietary intakes were standardized so that 40–45 percent of their calories came from carbohydrates. Patients in the study were asked to maintain their medications throughout the dietary and drug phases of the trial. On admission and at three-week intervals throughout the study, their fasting glucose and triglycerides serum values were evaluated, their food record was analyzed, their body mass index was measured, and their symptoms were recorded. Then, after the initial dietary phase, subjects were randomly assigned to receive either a placebo capsule or 200 milligrams of blueberry leaves extract powder in capsule form three times a day (taken with water before meals). During the initial period of diet counseling,

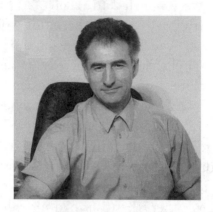

Professor Musa T. Abidoff, M.D., of the Moscow Center for Modern Medicine. Professor Abidoff has performed clinical studies using *Rhododendron caucasicum* extract, Caucasian blueberry leaves extract, and *Rhodiola rosea* extract

neither group experienced significant changes in fasting blood glucose values. However, beginning in week six of the trial's drug phase and continuing to the end of the trial, those individuals taking the blueberry leaves extract showed a significant reduction in mean plasma glucose levels. Their levels decreased to an average 136 milligrams per deciliter from 169 milligrams per deciliter.

Science rediscovers an ancient folk medicine. Dr. Zakir Ramazanov, for one, is not surprised at the results of research on Caucasian blueberry leaves. He says, "The reasons for Caucasian blueberry leaves' use to treat diabetes in folk medicine and the extract's growing popularity among the informed public is no longer a scientific mystery. Results of these Russian studies indicate that Caucasian blueberry leaves extract can help regulate blood glucose levels in both healthy people and diabetics."

"Caucasian blueberry leaves extract is a safe, natural, potent source of critical chlorogenic and hydroxycinnamic acids, and it has a long and venerable history," Dr. Ramazanov continues. "It has an even more promising future in the maintenance of good health and in the long-term care of diabetics everywhere."[10]

Additional Health Solutions

While Caucasian blueberry leaves extract is best known for preventing and treating sugar imbalances, modern research has shown that the extract has many additional and equally impressive health-protecting benefits. Among these benefits, Caucasian blueberry leaves extract has been shown to inhibit free radical damage, inhibit brain degeneration, protect the liver, minimize pesticide and radiation damage, and inhibit viruses. Most notably, in clinical studies the extract has also been shown to reduce levels of bad cholesterol and triglycerides in the body. Reducing these levels subsequently slows the onset and progression of atherosclerois (hardening of the arteries with buildup of plaque on the interior walls of arteries), and reduces the potential for heart attacks and strokes. All of these benefits, and others, slow the aging process and allow people to live happier, healthier, and longer lives.

CARDIOVASCULAR DISEASE

The American Heart Association estimates that more than 67 million Americans currently suffer from one or more cardiovascular diseases, and almost 950,000 Americans die each year from these diseases. Of those 950,000 cardiovascular deaths per year, approximately 440,000 are the result of heart attacks and 158,000 are the result of strokes.[51,52,53] The cost of health care and lost productivity due to cardiovascular disease is estimated to have totaled about $351 billion in 2003.[54]

While cardiovascular disease may result from various causes, it often is associated with abnormally high cholesterol and triglyceride levels.[55,56,57] Because of this, I'll next explain cholesterol and triglycerides in more detail. Then we'll explore how Caucasian blueberry leaves extract can help prevent unhealthy amounts and certain types of these substances from accumulating in the body.

Cholesterol. Cholesterol has many functions and is essential to life. As an indispensable building block and component of cell membranes, it is found throughout the human organism. Among other functions, it is key in synthesizing vitamin D, bile salts (which help digest foods, especially fatty ones), and steroid hormones, including male and female sex hormones. The human liver synthesizes between 1,500 and 2,000 milligrams of new cholesterol each day, of which about 15 percent is absorbed from what we eat and drink.

Generally when we eat, fat from our foods is digested, combined with proteins to form large lipoprotein molecules, and transported to the liver. The fat is then processed and excreted as very low density lipoproteins (VLDLs), which transport triglycerides to various tissues—primarily to adipose (fat storage) tissue. After the triglycerides have been unloaded, residues of VLDLs convert into low density lipoproteins (LDLs), which contain 60 percent to 70 percent of total blood cholesterol. LDLs are also called bad cholesterol because they can play the most deadly role in the formation of arterial plaque.[58-63]

LDLs cause a problem when one has too much of them in the blood and/or when they oxidize too fast. When this is the case, a series of cellular events allow the LDLs to attach to and then penetrate arterial walls, where immune system white blood cells, called macrophages, begin absorbing the cholesterol. The macrophages become engorged with the LDLs and convert into macrophage foam cells. These foam cells attract other blood cells, which continue the engorgement process. Over time, arterial plaque, which is mostly composed of LDLs, forms and then enlarges, and the arterial wall becomes progressively corrupt.[59-72]

Like other bodily components, cholesterol is subject to free radical damage, or damage from oxidation. And unfortunately, research now shows that LDLs modified by oxidation are absorbed at an advanced rate, which accelerates the formation of plaque.[62-72] To make matters worse, LDLs can also be oxidized by the very macrophage cells that absorb them.[72,73,74]

Fortunately, the body has a natural way to govern levels of LDL cholesterol. It involves high density lipoproteins (HDLs), or good cholesterol. HDLs help control LDL levels by scavenging LDLs from the walls of blood vessels and transporting them back to the liver for further processing and disposal.[59] Additionally, a substance called paraoxonase, which binds to HDLs, appears to protect both HDLs and LDLs from oxidation. However, both paraoxonase and HDLs can be rendered inactivated by oxidized lipids, including oxidized LDLs and oxidized HDLs.[75,76]

As mentioned, when one has too many LDLs in the blood or when LDLs oxidize too fast, cholesterol slowly builds in the arteries. Cholesterol buildup in the coronary arteries or the arteries that feed the brain leads to the formation of lesions composed of atherosclerotic plaque. This condition, called atherosclerosis, is the leading cause of death in the Western world.[10,77]

As atherosclerotic plaque lesions enlarge, they cause progressively serious damage to the body. They damage and destroy local arterial tissue and can reduce blood flow in the affected arteries. This reduction in blood flow means that the tissues the arteries supply, including heart, brain, and other tissues, receive less blood and nutrients. And obviously, as the arterial passageways become progressively smaller, they can be blocked by correspondingly smaller blood clots—clumps composed of blood cells, bacteria, parasites, dead tissue, scar tissue, calcium, cholesterol, fat globules, yeast, or gas bubbles. As a blockage increases, clumps that may have passed undeterred through normal arteries can, in atherosclerotic arteries, block blood flow to the heart and cause a heart attack or block blood flow to the brain and cause a stroke.[78]

Other physiological factors, including additional free radical damage, genetics, infections, hypertension, and chemical interactions, facilitate the build up of atherosclerotic plaque.[79] Nonetheless a key factor in atherosclerotic plaque buildup is bad cholesterol—especially oxidized bad cholesterol. Atherosclerotic plaque is rich in cholesterol, and the more LDLs there are in the blood, the faster the disease begins and advances.[60] Therefore, the primary keys to controlling the onset and progression of atherosclerosis are to limit LDLs to safe levels and to protect LDLs and HDLs from oxidation—without causing additional problems.

Triglycerides. Like cholesterol, triglycerides are small fat molecules essential to life. While cholesterol is a building block for cells, triglycerides provide much of the energy cells need to function. Triglycerides join with fatty acids and protein to form the lipoproteins called VLDLs. These lipoproteins travel through the bloodstream, depositing triglycerides in the body's cells.[60]

The problem occurs when the level of triglycerides in the

Table 11. Cholesterol and Triglyceride Levels

Total Cholesterol

Desirable blood cholesterol	Less than 200 mg/dl
Borderline-high blood cholesterol	200 to 239 mg/dl
High blood cholesterol	240 mg/dl and higher

Source: American Heart Association. 2004.[84]

LDL ("bad") Cholesterol

Optimal LDL blood cholesterol	Less than 100 mg/dl
Borderline high LDL blood cholesterol	130 to 159 mg/dl
High LDL blood cholesterol	160 to 189 mg/dl
Very high LDL blood cholesterol	190 mg/dl and higher

Source: ATP III. 2001. American Heart Association. 2004.[84]

HDL ("good") Cholesterol

Low HDL blood cholesterol	Less than 40 mg/dl
High HDL blood cholesterol	60 mg/dl and higher

Source: American Heart Association. 2004.[84]

Triglycerides

Normal triglycerides	Less than 150 mg/dl
Borderline-high triglycerides	150 to 199 mg/dl
High triglycerides	200 to 499 mg/dl
Very high triglycerides	Greater than 500 mg/dl

Source: ATP III. 2001. American Heart Association. 2004.[85]

blood gets too high. The dangers of high triglyceride levels can be found in the results of epidemiological research. Professor Melissa A. Austin of the University of Washington led a twenty-year study to examine, through medical histories, the LDL and triglyceride levels of 685 members of 101 families. The research revealed that family members with elevated triglyceride levels were two to three times more likely to die from cardiovascular disease than those whose triglyceride levels were normal—even when the family members with high triglyceride levels had normal LDL levels.[80] And in addition to increasing the likelihood of cardiovascular disease, exceedingly high triglyceride levels can also cause the pancreas gland to become inflamed. This condition, called pancreatitis, can be quite debilitating. Severe, acute pancreatitis can result in death.[81]

For future reference, the most common cholesterol measurement is a test for total cholesterol; in fact, when describing their cholesterol levels as 139, 183, 247, or 395, most people are referring to their total cholesterol levels. Total cholesterol is the sum of all five known lipoproteins: chylomicrons, LDLs, HDLs, VLDLs, and IDLs (intermediate density lipoproteins).[82] According to the American Heart Association, an estimated 102.3 million American adults have total blood cholesterol levels of 200 or higher, and an estimated 41.3 million American adults have total blood cholesterol levels of 240 or higher.[83]

Cholesterol- and triglyceride-lowering drugs. Obviously, when patients' cholesterol and triglyceride levels get too high, doctors look to drugs to reduce these levels. And as a matter of fact, scientific studies indicate that these anticholesterol drugs are very effective at treating hypercholesterolemia. However, these same drugs simultaneously reduce the amount of vitamin E in the blood. They also reduce the levels of very important compounds such as coenzyme Q10, an essential mitochondrial energy-producing component and antioxidant, and levels of the important amino acid-like substance L-carnitine.[86-91] Therefore, it would be better for the body if a method of reducing cholesterol without side effects could be found.

Phenolics and cholesterol reduction. As previously stated, research shows that arterial macrophage foam cells absorb oxidation-modified LDLs at an advanced rate, which thereby quickens the formation of arterial plaque. Therefore, the goal of any cholesterol treatment should be to safely reduce LDL levels while simultaneously limiting LDL oxidation. With this in mind, one possible solution for safely reducing LDL levels and limiting LDL oxidation is to use natural herbal formulations rather than purified pharmaceuticals. Fruits and vegetables, for instance, which are rich in antioxidants, have been used effectively throughout the world to treat many conditions, including high blood cholesterol and circulatory conditions.[3,10]

Caucasian blueberry leaves may also be effective in this regard, thanks to their high levels of the antioxidants chlorogenic acid and hydroxycinnamic acid. This is because, based on various studies, it is evident that these antioxidants significantly reduce LDL levels and provide a great deal of protection against LDL oxidation while also maintaining, and even enhancing, the amount of vitamin E in the blood.[92-96]

One study reported in the *Archives of Biochemistry and Biophysics* that supplementing rats' diets with hydroxycinnamic acid resulted in a statistically significant increase of vitamin E in both plasma and lipoprotein. LDLs in hydroxycinnamic acid-fed rats were also more resistant to oxidation. These results clearly demonstrate hydroxycinnamic acid's antioxidant action.[96]

The significance of hydroxycinnamic acid's ability to maintain healthy levels of vitamin E in our bodies should not be underestimated. Hydroxycinnamic acid preserves vitamin E

Table 12. Caucasian Blueberry Leaves: Lipid Study 1

Beginning of Study: Prior to Blueberry Leaves Applications
Mean Plasma Lipid Levels

LDL ("Bad" Cholesterol)	141
Triglycerides	179

End of Study: After Blueberry Leaves Applications
Mean Plasma Lipid Levels

LDL ("Bad" Cholesterol)	115
Triglycerides	130

Source: Musa T. Abidoff, M.D., 1999.[2]

when it is present before the vitamin E is challenged by free radicals and toxins. Hydroxycinnamic acid also restores vitamin E when added halfway through the oxidation process. And in LDLs enriched with vitamin E, hydroxycinnamic acid recycles good vitamin E from the vitamin E radical.[10]

Blueberry leaves extract, triglycerides, and cholesterol. Beyond the positive effects of the chlorogenic and hydroxycinnamic acids contained in Caucasian blueberry leaves, science has also shown that Caucasian blueberry leaves extract can lower cholesterol and triglyceride levels.

In one animal study—the aforementioned Italian research that determined the therapeutic action of blueberry leaves extract on diabetes—scientists measured the extract's effectiveness at lowering triglyceride levels. They administered blueberry leaves extract to streptozotocin-diabetic rats for four days. In the end (and as previously mentioned), blood sugar levels decreased 26 percent. But in addition, and to the surprise of the researchers, plasma triglyceride also decreased—by 39 percent—following treatment.[47] These findings indicate that blueberry leaves' active constituents may prove useful for treating certain instances of high triglycerides.

Blueberry leaves extract was also shown to affect triglyceride and cholesterol levels in another previously mentioned study, this one by the Russian scientist Musa Abidoff, M.D. As you will recall, his clinical trial measured the effects of Caucasian blueberry leaves extract on Type 2 diabetics' glucose levels. Subjects received either a placebo or 200 milligrams of Caucasian blueberry leaves extract powder in capsule form three times a day (taken with water before meals). By the end of the study, the triglyceride levels of those taking the blueberry leaves extract had dropped to an average 130 milligrams per deciliter from 179 milligrams per deciliter. In addition, LDL values in these patients dropped to an average 115 milligrams per deciliter from 141 milligrams per deciliter.[2]

Additional protection from cardiovascular disease. To review, high LDL (bad cholesterol), high oxidized LDL, and high triglyceride levels are major risk factors for cardiovascular disease, and Caucasian blueberry leaves extract has been shown to help keep these substances in check. However, there are other causes of cardiovascular disease and heart failure. Fortunately, Caucasian blueberry leaves extract is also effective against some of these as well. Most notably, Caucasian blueberry leaves extract's two most voluminous constituents, chlorogenic acid and hydroxycinnamic acid, inhibit a heart-disease-promoting free radical molecule called peroxynitrite.

Peroxynitrite is toxic to cells, and increasingly, it is being called a contributor to tissue injury in several human diseases, including heart disease, multiple sclerosis, Parkinson's disease, and Alzheimer's disease.[97-100] Peroxynitrite can react to a wide range of molecules to damage cells through peroxidation, oxidation, and nitration. It also adversely reacts to two key proteins necessary for healthy heart contraction. Detection of nitrotyrosine, a by-product of peroxynitrite, in inflamed tissue serves as a marker of damage caused by peroxynitrite. As reported in the journal *Critical Care Medicine*, heart tissue obtained from patients with myocarditis (inflammation of the middle muscle layer of the heart wall) and sepsis (pus-forming infections) has "significantly higher" levels of nitrotyrosine than non-diseased heart tissue.[97]

The good news is that numerous studies have shown that chlorogenic acid and hydroxycinnamic acid, as are found in Caucasian blueberry leaves, are two of the most powerful natural inhibitors of peroxynitrite. For example, research performed at Argentina's University of Buenos Aires and published in the *Annals of the New York Academy of Sciences* reports that chlorogenic and hydroxycinnamic acids ". . . were effective inhibitors of the [peroxynitrite] ONOO(-)-driven oxidation reactions."[101] Research performed at Portugal's University of Coimbra and published in *Free Radical Research* reports that chlorogenic and hydroxycinnamic acids "inhibit" the oxidation of LDL and loss of vitamin E [triggered by peroxynitrite].[102] And research performed at Japan's Shimane University and published in *Biochimica et Biophysica Acta* reports that ". . . chlorogenic acid inhibited the initiation of chain lipid peroxidations by organic free radical [peroxynitrite]."[103]

Thus, by inhibiting peroxynitrite and other free radicals, and by lowering cholesterol and triglyceride levels, Caucasian blueberry leaves extract effectively helps prevent cardiovascular diseases. And as noted above, the extract is also useful in fighting other illnesses.

PARKINSON'S DISEASE AND BRAIN DEGENERATION

Parkinson's disease is the most common neurodegenerative disease after Alzheimer's. It afflicts more people than multiple sclerosis, muscular dystrophy, and Lou Gehrig's disease combined. According to the National Parkinson's Foundation, as many as 1.5 million Americans suffer from Parkinson's disease,[104] and the Parkinson's Action Network estimates that about 60,000 new cases are diagnosed yearly.[105] The economic toll of Parkinson's Disease on American society is estimated to be as high as $25 billion per year.[106,107]

Parkinson's disease is a progressively debilitating illness. Its symptoms include a decrease in the spontaneity and speed of movement, rigidity, pain, muscle cramps, dementia, difficulty swallowing, and usually a resting tremor. These symptoms result when certain neurons in the midbrain die. These neurons produce the neurotransmitter dopamine.[107–109]

One of the biggest problems Parkinson's researchers and clinicians have, according to Dr. A. H. V. Schapira, professor of clinical neurosciences at University College London, is that "by the time patients' symptoms become sufficiently apparent for them to seek help, about 70 to 80 percent of their dopaminergic neurons [the brain cells that produce the neurotransmitter dopamine] may already have died."[109] Thus, as Dr. Schapira continues, the main challenges in treating Parkinson's disease are: "(1) to protect dopaminergic neurons so that either the disease is prevented or its progression is slowed, and (2) to provide early treatment to 'rescue' neurons at risk."[109]

Of course, knowing how to protect these neurons requires knowing what causes them to be damaged. According to Dr.

Zakir Ramazanov, "There is some evidence that inflammatory processes and peroxynitrite radicals may play a role in nerve cell [neuron] damage in Parkinson's disease. Peroxynitrite has long been known to be a strong oxidant. Prolonged exposure to peroxynitrite may impair mechanisms in body fluids [that] defend against peroxynitrite and other free radicals, resulting in increased tissue sensitivity to oxidative damage."[3,10]

The good news is that, again, Caucasian blueberry leaves extract may help prevent nerve cell [neuron] damage, thanks to its ability to inhibit peroxynitrite. In a study reported in the *Journal of Neuroscience*, Drs. N. Kerry and C. Rice-Evans of King's College London investigated the interaction between peroxynitrite and dopamine, and how antioxidants might inhibit this interaction. They found that peroxynitrite promoted dopamine oxidation, which would damage nerve cells. However, they also found that hydroxycinnamic acid, as found in Caucasian blueberry leaves extract, inhibited the dopamine oxidation caused by peroxynitrite.[110] These findings suggest that consuming fruit-based phenolic compounds, such as the hydroxycinnamic and chlorogenic acids found in abundance in Caucasian blueberry leaves extract, can inhibit dopamine oxidation and protect neurotransmitters from peroxynitrite-induced depletion. Or in other words, Caucasian blueberry leaves may prove useful against Parkinson's disease.

ADDITIONAL NEURODEGENERATIVE PROCESSES

An enzyme called 5-lipoxygenase was recently discovered in the brain's neuronal cells, and scientists at the Psychiatric Institute of the University of Illinois, Chicago, have learned that it multiplies in these cells as we age. This increase can injure the neuronal cells and cause them to leak fluid and die.[111-113]

Fortunately, the scientists also found that hydroxycinnamic acid could inhibit 5-lipoxygenase and thereby protect against neurodegeneration.[113] Thus, since hydroxycinnamic acid is a key component of Caucasian blueberry leaves extract, the extract is also a promising 5-lipoxygenase inhibitor. It can play a key role in supporting healthy brain functions and slowing neurodegeneration.

In addition to the enzyme 5-lipoxygenase, low density lipoproteins (LDLs), or bad cholesterol, also exist within the brain. LDLs are highly vulnerable to oxidation by toxins and free radicals. Once oxidized, they are capable of inflaming non-neuronal brain cells and killing the neuronal cells of the central nervous system.[114-116] As Drs. H. Schroeter, R. J. Williams, R. Matin, L. Iversen, and C. A. Rice-Evans of King's College London have demonstrated, oxidized LDLs enter neuronal cells and cause DNA fragmentation, cell breakdown, and cell death.[117]

However, these scientists' research has also demonstrated that flavonoids, hydroxycinnamic acid derivatives (but in this case not hydroxycinnamic acid itself), and hydroxycinnamic acid compounds, including chlorogenic acid, reduce neuronal loss—the loss associated with neurodegenerative disorders such as Alzheimer's disease and Parkinson's disease. "Because of the observed protective effects of phenolic antioxidants in this study," the scientists wrote in the journal *Free Radical Biology and Medicine*, "we propose that these compounds do not act solely as antioxidants, but might interact with downstream signaling events . . . that lead ultimately to neuronal cell death. In summary, flavonoids and hydroxycinnamic acid derivatives demonstrate potent neuroprotective actions . . . which could have important implications for the potential use of these compounds against neuronal loss observed in . . . neurodegenerative diseases and cognitive declines associated with aging."[117] In other words, hydroxycinnamic acid derivatives and chlorogenic acid, as found in Caucasian blueberry leaves extract, could potentially slow or stop the neural cell damage associated with brain degeneration.

CANCER

Most nitrosamines are carcinogens—toxic compounds that cause various cancers. They lead to cancer of the liver, stomach, bladder, and other organs. In fact, of the approximately 300 different nitrosamines that have been evaluated, more than 90 percent have been found to induce cancer. These carcinogens can cause acute poisoning and death. In addition, they can interact with the central nervous system to cause fluid buildup in the brain, which can cause lethargy, confusion, incontinence, nausea, vomiting, severe headaches, seizures, visual impairment, irritability, tiredness, hallucinations, and sometimes coma.[118-122]

Nitrosamines appear in the foods we eat, especially those high in nitrites, such as cured meats.[123] This might explain why a 1980-1987 study of children age ten and younger in Los Angeles County found that children who ate more that twelve hot dogs a month were nine times more likely to develop childhood leukemia.[124] However, although approximately 39 percent of dietary nitrite intake comes from bacon, ham, sausage, and other cured meats, research shows that 34 percent of nitrites are consumed through baked goods and cereals and 16 percent are consumed through vegetables. Nitrites are also in the water we drink, although levels vary widely from area to area.[125,126]

Additionally, tobacco smoke contains specific nitrosamines that have been linked to cancer.[127] The National Academy of Sciences estimates that smokers' exposure to volatile nitrosamines through cigarettes is 200 times higher than the nitrosamine exposure one would get from eating bacon every day—and bacon is the food with the highest nitrosamine levels.[128]

Now, researchers have found that consuming a significant amount of chlorogenic acid might prevent nitrosamines from forming. As reported in the *Biochemical Journal*, chlorogenic acid, a primary constituent of Caucasian blueberry leaves extract, is a strong inhibitor of nitrosamines. It is also very effective at inhibiting chemical reactions that could potentially cause genetic mutations and cancer.[129,130] Scientific studies also suggest that chlorogenic acid may help prevent stomach cancer.[131,132] Again, this is because, in addition to its ability to inhibit nitrosamine formation, chlorogenic acid can protect DNA from free radical damage.[133]

In using chlorogenic acid against nitrosamines, it appears that significant amounts of this special phenolic antioxidant must be consumed. That's where Caucasian blueberry leaves extract comes in. Because Caucasian blueberry leaves extract contains large amounts of chlorogenic acid, it may provide an effective first line of defense against the development of cancer.

HERBICIDE POISONING

Most Americans regularly consume foods contaminated with herbicides and pesticides.[134-137] In fact, a 2002 study led by the Consumers Union found pesticide residue on 75 percent of conventionally grown fruits and vegetables, and on 23 percent of organically grown fruits and vegetables. These included long-banned pesticides such as DDT.[138]

Paraquat is another widely used herbicide that is highly toxic to both animals and humans. Sometimes referred to as "one of the dirty dozen,"[139] it can damage the heart, lungs, gas-

trointestinal tract, kidneys, and liver—with significant exposure—by inducing oxidation. In other words, paraquat generates powerful free radicals.[140-145]

Fortunately, chlorogenic acid, as found in abundance in
Caucasian blueberry leaves extract, has been shown to prevent paraquat from damaging body tissues. Researchers at
Japan's Yamagata University examined chlorogenic acid's
protective effects against paraquat-induced oxidative stress,
or free radical damage. In this controlled study, a group of rats
was fed a diet that included paraquat. As expected, the
paraquat produced huge increases in free radical damage and
changes in blood chemistry that are indicative of tissue damage and disease. However, when chlorogenic acid was added
to the rats' diet, all indicators of oxidative stress, tissue damage, and disease returned to normal levels. The rats' food
intake and weight gain also normalized.[146]

RADIATION DAMAGE

Gamma rays and X-rays are very similar forms of high-
energy radiation.[147] Sufficient exposure to these rays causes
DNA damage, scrambling of the genetic code, brain tumors,
and cancer, including leukemia.[148-153] However, chlorogenic
acid, one of the two primary constituents of Caucasian blueberry leaves, has been shown to limit the damage such radiation produces.

Drs. S. K. Abraham, L. Sarma, and P. C. Kesavan of India's
Jawaharlal Nehru University studied what effect chlorogenic
acid might have in preventing DNA damage in mice that had
been subjected to gamma radiation. They found that by giving the mice chlorogenic acid (in doses of 50, 100, or 200 milligrams per 2.2 pounds of body weight), they could "significantly" reduce the amount of DNA damage caused by

gamma-radiation exposure. The scientists observed less DNA damage after administering just one dose of the phenolic, given two hours before the radiation exposure or immediately after it. They also observed less damage to bone marrow cells in samples taken 24, 30, and 48 hours after radiation exposure.[154] The results of this study indicate that chlorogenic acid, one of the most voluminous components of Caucasian blueberry leaves extract, may provide significant protection against the damaging effects of radiation.

HERPES

Approximately 80 to 90 percent of the U.S. population over fifty years of age is infected with herpes simplex virus Type 1, or oral herpes, and approximately 22 percent of American adults are infected with herpes simplex virus Type 2, or genital herpes.[155,156,157] Sadly, less than 10 percent of Americans who test positive for genital herpes and are capable of transmitting the disease to others are aware they are infected, and as many as 1 million Americans become infected with this type of herpes each year.[158,159] Canadian researchers have even projected that 49 percent of all American women and 39 percent of all American men between the ages of 15 and 39 will be infected with genital herpes by the year 2025.[160]

People infected with either type of herpes have far more to worry about than outbreaks of sores. Recent research indicates that those infected with Type 1 herpes may be predisposed to developing Alzheimer's disease.[161,162] Also, Type 1 herpes sufferers who are at least 65 years old are two times more likely to die from heart disease than those who are not infected.[163] And finally, women suffering from Type 2 genital herpes have an increased risk of developing cervical cancer.[164,165,166]

The good news is that Caucasian blueberry leaves may help. For many centuries, these leaves (along with *Rhododendron caucasicum* and Georgian pomegranate) have been used in folk medicine to treat infections, and now, modern research has verified that the leaves' primary constituents exhibit strong antiviral activity.[167-173] Specifically, German Dr. K. D. Thiel and his colleagues have demonstrated that hydroxycinnamic acid, which is found in abundance in Caucasian blueberry leaves, is effective at fighting both herpes simplex virus type 1 and type 2. Dr. Thiel's team found that hydroxycinnamic acid's effectiveness against herpes was higher during the early phase of the infection. However, the phenolic was active even seventy-two hours after virus absorption.[126] Based on Dr. Thiel's findings, Caucasian blueberry leaves extract may offer effective prevention against and treatment for herpes.

HUMAN IMMUNODEFICIENCY VIRUS (HIV)

More than 40 million people worldwide are infected with HIV, the virus that causes AIDS. In addition, sixty thousand Americans become infected with HIV each year. The virus has caused between 13 million and 20 million deaths worldwide, and the United Nations predicts that an additional 68 million to 70 million people will die from AIDS within the next eighteen years unless there are dramatic lifestyles changes and improvements in AIDS prevention and treatment.[174-176]

HIV kills by damaging the immune system. Normally, the system's CD4 cells (also called T-helper cells) protect the body from infections and diseases, but when HIV enters the body, it infects and destroys these CD4 cells. This dramatically impairs the immune system's ability to fight other infections and diseases. Thus, many infections that could be destroyed by a healthy immune system become deadly for those with HIV.[177]

Fortunately, leading researchers have now demonstrated that hydroxycinnamic acid and chlorogenic acid derivatives appear to inhibit HIV, as crude extracts containing these phenolic acids—the two key components of Caucasian blueberry leaves extract—have shown strong HIV-fighting activity.[178] Scientists at the University of California, Irvine, have shown that several hydroxycinnamic and chlorogenic acid derivatives, namely dicaffeoylquinic acids and two analogues, were potent and selective inhibitors of HIV in vitro. They also found that all chlorogenic acid derivatives could inhibit HIV replication.[179] These results and others indicate that chlorogenic acid and hydroxycinnamic acid derivatives are important HIV inhibitors and may form crucial lead compounds in the development of HIV drugs.[180–182] Additionally, the results are one more proof of the value of Caucasian blueberry leaves extract, which has now been shown to have the potential to protect the body from myriad illnesses.

Choosing a Caucasian Blueberry Leaf Extract

The benefits that Caucasian blueberry leaves provide for sufferers of diabetes and other sugar imbalances are legendary. Research also documents Caucasian blueberry leaves extract's effectiveness at lowering bad cholesterol and triglyceride levels. And now, additional research has demonstrated the tremendous protection Caucasian blueberry leaves extract's two key constituents, chlorogenic acid and hydroxycinnamic acid, provide against a score of other dangerous ills. Truly, Caucasian blueberry leaves extract can provide consumers with unparalleled defenses against many illnesses and aging.

At the same time, consumers should be aware that only Caucasian blueberry leaves extract can produce the benefits just described. Fifty years of research has demonstrated that the extract's protective and healing effects depend on several factors, including what species of plant was used, where the plants were grown, and how the nutrients were extracted. Varying any one of these factors can bring far less than satisfying results. In addition, positive results can only be obtained from consuming products made from Caucasian blueberry leaves, not from berries, blueberries, or even common blueberry leaves.

KEY FACTORS IN EFFECTIVENESS

The three factors that ensure Caucasian blueberry leaves extract's effectiveness are the species used to produce the extract, the methods by which the plants are cultivated and harvested, and the way in which the plant's beneficial chemicals are extracted.

The species of plant is particularly important. There are, in fact, about twenty-four recognized species of blueberry plants, and their phytochemical compositions vary. Therefore, the only way to ensure that an extract has the highest levels of beneficial phenolics is to look for one made specifically from either the plant species *Vaccinium arctostaphylos L*, or Georgian high-altitude *Vaccinium myrtillus L.*

Methods of cultivation and extraction are also important. It is common practice for blueberry plants to be sprayed with pesticides. Furthermore, Western methods of extracting beneficial chemicals from blueberry plants almost always include the use of toxic organic solvents, which remain as residue in end products. Both pesticides and toxic organic solvents produce powerful free radicals that are harmful to the human organism.

On the other hand, the Caucasian blueberry plant grows wild in the herbicide-free soil of Georgia's Caucasus Mountains and are never exposed to pesticides. Moreover, its nutrients are extracted using water and ethyl alcohol, not toxic organic solvents. Therefore, Caucasian blueberry leaves extract is free of the harmful residues that often appear in other extracts.

BEYOND BLUEBERRIES AND BLUEBERRY LEAVES

Why blueberry leaves? Why not the blueberries themselves, or berries in general? Well, as you might guess, blueberries (and all berries) contain natural sugar, which increases rather than decreases glucose levels and which can increase cholesterol and triglyceride levels. Caucasian blueberry leaves do not contain sugar and can therefore provide benefits without any drawbacks. In addition, Caucasian blueberry plants have been studied and analyzed for decades at the Georgian Academy of Sciences, and the research has consistently shown that the plants' most beneficial phytonutrient compounds are found in the leaves.[5]

Why Caucasian blueberry leaves extract? Why not common blueberry leaves? As mentioned, phenolic amounts vary from species to species in blueberry plants. Common blueberry leaves provide only about 1/60 of the phenolic volume of standardized Caucasian blueberry leaves extract. But also, common blueberry plants' growth at low altitudes and the standard processing practices of harvesting the berries prior to the leaves, using mature leaves, using pesticide in cultivation, and using toxic solvents in processing and extraction would render any extract made from common blueberry leaves inferior to Caucasian blueberry leaves extract. Such plant products would not and could not produce the results that have been detailed and verified through scientific research in this book. [3,10]

Caucasian blueberry leaves extract is standardized to contain precise amounts of beneficial phenolics. Only leaves from two species of Caucasian blueberry plants are harvested for use: *Vaccinium arctostaphylos L*, and Georgian high-altitude *Vaccinium myrtillus L*. Both of these species grow in the wild at high altitudes and have been analyzed in laboratory research. And as previously mentioned, these plants' phenolics are extracted without the use of toxic organic solvents. In addition, only young spring leaves are harvested for use in the extract. This is because young leaves contain much higher levels of chlorogenic and hydroxycinnamic acids than mature leaves. Finally, the leaves are harvested first, before the berries are formed, which further ensures maximum phenolic content.

Based on the aforementioned, and for reasons of both effectiveness and value, consumers should be sure that any blueberry leaves product meets the following specifications (which match the conditions used in the clinical studies on diabetes and cholesterol control):

- The product is made from one or both of two Caucasian blueberry leaves species: *Vaccinium arctosaphylos L,* or Georgian high-altitude *Vaccinium myrtillus L.*
- The plants used in the product grew at high altitudes on the Caucasus Mountains in the republic of Georgia.
- The plants' leaves were harvested in the spring, when they were young.
- The plants grew in the wild without the use of herbicides or pesticides.
- The plants' leaves were harvested before the berries were formed.

• The product does not contain toxic solvents.
• The product meets the standard of containing at least 20 percent chlorogenic and hydroxycinnamic acids.

Ancient Wisdom, Modern Science

Like *Rhododendron caucasicum*, Caucasian blueberry leaves' safety and benefits have been demonstrated by long-living Georgians for more than 2,000 years. In addition, the plant has been used in Georgian folk medicine for more than 600 years. Now, science has caught up with folk medicine. In clinical studies, Caucasian blueberry leaves extract, which contains two very important phenolic antioxidants, has proved effective against a host of ills. That's why Caucasian blueberry leaves are one of four key components of the Georgian diet described in this book.

Next, we'll discuss a third important Georgian plant: the Georgian pomegranate.

CHAPTER 5

Georgian Pomegranate

Pomegranate (*Punica granatum L*), the well-known fruit filled with myriad juicy seeds, is native to areas of the Middle East, the Caucasus, and the northern coast of Africa, but it has been widely dispersed throughout the centuries. Today its different versions of varying chemistries are found at warm latitudes around the world. Pomegranate now also grows throughout the southern United States, and it can thrive outdoors as far north as Washington, D. C.[1,2,3] The name *pomegranate* is believed by most to come from the Latin words for "apple" (*pomum*) and "full-of-seeds" (*granatus*). Others believe the name is derived from an earlier Latin name for the fruit, *Malum punicum*, which translates to "Carthaginian apple."[4,1] In either case, pomegranate has held an interesting place in history.

Ancient Assyrians and Egyptians held pomegranate sacred and frequently incorporated elaborate pomegranate carvings into architectural designs.[5] Pomegranates were also grown in

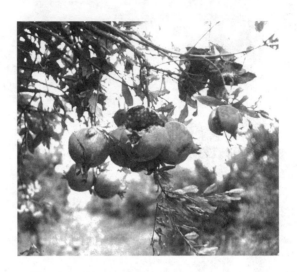

Pomegranates hanging in a grove

the hanging gardens of Babylon, which were built sometime between 810 B.C. and 562 B.C. And when Xerxes and other Persian kings traveled to battle fronts, they rode in royal chariots surrounded by elite troops, and these troops were followed by 10,000 "immortals," each of whom carried lances topped with golden pomegranates.[6] In Jerusalem, two freestanding columns with capitals decorated in pomegranates stood at the entrance to the Temple of Solomon, which was completed in 952 B.C. [7] Additionally, the temple's high priest wore a robe with a hem of embroidered pomegranates in blue, purple, and scarlet, separated by gold bells.[8] The Old Testament lists pomegranate as one of five fruits with which the promised land of Israel was blessed.[9,10]

Pomegranate has also been popular in Georgia and the Caucasus—this time as a key dietary component. Traditional Georgian salads are made from green onions, wild garlic, nettle leaves, watercress, basil, parsley, cilantro, dill, and tomato, but even more important, they are dressed with ground walnut, horse chestnuts, and pomegranate. Also, traditional Georgian cuisine is particularly rich in sauces made from plums, blackberries, blueberries, grapes, and pomegranates, along with fermented milk (matzoni/kefir/yogurt), garlic, and vegetables. Finally, pomegranate juice is a favorite Georgian treat, and both pomegranate juice and pomegranate seeds are used in meat dressings.[11]

But in addition to the pomegranate's cultural and dietary history, the fruit has an interesting medicinal history as well.

Medicinal History of the Pomegranate

Pomegranate's use as a medicine reaches back into time immemorial.[12] In fact, pomegranate was first mentioned in the papyrus *Ebers of Egypt*, which includes medicinal information collected from as far back as 3,550 B.C.[13] Later, in about 377 B.C., Hippocrates described pomegranate's medicinal power. And by 77 A.D., the Greek physician Dioscorides had described pomegranate's medicinal properties in his masterpiece *De Materia Medica*.[5]

How was pomegranate used? Historically, doctors in Greece have prescribed its juice as a remedy for multiple ills. They used this juice as an anti-inflammatory, as a potent antihelmintic (a substance that destroys certain intestinal worms), and as a cough suppressant. They also found it to be effective against chronic diarrhea and dysentery. In Georgian and Mediterranean folk medicines, pomegranate was used to arrest chronic mucous discharges, passive hemorrhages, night sweats, and diarrhea. Pomegranate was also employed to strengthen human capillaries and to prevent atherosclerosis, asthma, tonsillitis, and bronchitis. In addition, as Dr. Zakir Ramazanov has noted, pomegranate extract mixed with aloe extract has been used to activate bone tissue regeneration after injury.[11] And from 1948 to 1950, Georgian scientist Alaristakh Mshvidovandze, Ph.D., conducted intensive research into the healing properties of pomegranate and found that the fruit also could be made into a successful burn treatment.[14]

Besides the aforementioned uses, pomegranate has been employed in other medicinal ways. In many cultures, pomegranate has traditionally been used to treat the pain associated with parasitic infections and to treat rectal prolapse, involuntary rectal emissions, and bleeding during bowel movements. Interestingly, it has also been used as an aphrodisiac. In addition, one pomegranate constituent, pelleterine, has proven to be effective against tapeworms (but not other intestinal parasites); the pomegranate alkaloids cause the tapeworm to relax its grip on the intestinal wall, which makes it possible for the tapeworm to be expelled by cathartics.[15] And last but not least, pomegranate is an ingredient in a remedy for dysentery and chronic diarrhea, and its rind is used in postpartum medication.

Today, pomegranate is destined to become quite famous in medicine again. This is because it contains extremely high volumes of the anticancer phenolic ellagic acid, and because it is very active in fighting cardiovascular diseases.[11,16,17] Next, we'll explore the Georgian pomegranate's anticancer properties in more detail by examining what causes various cancers and how the ellagic acid in Georgian pomegranate might help prevent and treat the disease.

Cancer

Cancer is a prominent killer, second only to heart disease. It currently causes one out of every four deaths in the United

States, and the American Cancer Society estimates that during 2003 cancer took the lives of 556,500 Americans—more than 1,524 people per day. Also during 2004, about 1,334,100 new cancer cases are expected to be diagnosed in the United States. Over time, one of every two men and one of every three women will likely develop cancer. All told, the cost of cancer-related treatments, lost wages, lost productivity, and losses associated with premature death due to cancer during 2002 was estimated at $171.6 billion.[18,19]

What exactly is cancer? For starters, the term "cancer" defines more than 100 separate diseases, and all are related to cell production.[20] More specifically, with cancer, the body's natural method of producing cells is corrupted. But let's step back just a little for some background.

The human body is composed of some 100 trillion cells, which routinely reproduce themselves by dividing—a process called mitosis. Through mitosis, cells that are damaged, diseased, worn out, dead, or lost due to injuries are replaced with new cells. The process is regulated, so the body only reproduces enough cells to perform the duties required for maintaining good health. And in a perfect world, that regulated process and orderly growth and repair of body tissues would continue throughout a lifetime.

A problem can occur, though, and often does, when the mechanisms that regulate a cell's rate of mitosis are damaged. Suddenly, the cell is free to reproduce itself without inner restraint. The single damaged cell divides, producing an equally damaged and dangerous clone of itself. Then those two cells subsequently divide to create four, the four divide to create eight, the eight divide to create sixteen, and so on— true exponential growth. Over time, a lump, mass, or tumor forms.[18,21-23]

As William M. Rich, M.D., of the University of California

at San Francisco, explains, "The smallest lump, mass, or tumor that can be detected by physical examination, X-ray, or C.T. scan is a little less than a quarter-inch in diameter. An anomaly of that size would contain between 100 million to 1 billion cells. The smallest lump, mass, or tumor that can be detected by a mammogram would contain about 100 thousand to 1 million cells."[21,24] This means that it often takes ten or more years, from the instant the mitosis regulator in a cell is damaged, for cells to multiply into a mass large enough to be detected by common medical methods.[18,21,25] Therefore, as can be imagined, a frighteningly high percentage of us, reading this book at this moment, have tumors growing within us—even if we've recently received clean bills of health.

Tumors can be cancerous (malignant) or cancer-free (benign), and there are many differences between the two. The most apparent differences are that malignant tumors have an abnormal appearance, grow more rapidly than other tumors, and release their cancerous cells to other parts of the body where additional tumors form in a process called metastasis. Of course, benign tumors can and often do develop into malignant tumors over time.[23,26,27]

What causes cancer? An ever increasing number of chemicals, biological agents such as viruses and parasites, and physical agents such as ultraviolet light and radiation are being identified as carcinogens, or cancer-causing agents. Dietary factors, such as high fat intake, and chronic injuries and inflammations, such as scarring and pressure ulcers, have also been linked to cancer development. Michio Kaku, Ph.D., the renowned professor of theoretical physics at the City College of the City University of New York has said that "epidemiologists have determined that a vast majority, perhaps as many as 70 to 90 percent, of all cancers can be correlated to the environment and lifestyle."[28] In addition, genetic predispositions often greatly increase a person's chances of developing certain types of cancer. But in any event, when a single cell first begins to replicate at an abnormally high rate, it is the result of damage to the cell's DNA, or genetic instructions.[23,27,29,30] This damage most frequently occurs through the destructive work of free radicals.[31]

ELLAGIC ACID AND CANCER

Studies reveal that we are constantly exposed to cancer-causing agents. Many of these carcinogens remain within our bodies, posing a risk to our cells and DNA for decades.[32-36] Specific fruit and vegetable phenolics have been shown to inhibit free radical damage to cells and DNA caused by carcinogens. Therefore, these same phenolics should reduce the formation of certain cancers.[11,37]

As previously noted, chlorogenic and hydroxycinnamic acids are two of the most powerful phenolics in this regard.[38-41] Chlorogenic acid and hydroxycinnamic acid derivatives are found in abundance in *Rhododendron caucasicum* extract, and chlorogenic and hydroxycinnamic acids comprise at least 20 percent of Caucasian blueberry leaves extract. In addition, the Georgian pomegranate's ellagic acid is yet another powerful cancer inhibitor.

Interest in ellagic acid has increased during the last several years primarily because of its extraordinary effectiveness at protecting against genetic mutations and cancer. This effectiveness is revealed in several published scientific studies. For example, Dr. Gary Stoner of Ohio State University is one of the pioneering scientists who directed research that has clearly demonstrated ellagic acid's medicinal properties. Dr. Stoner's initial studies on rodents have shown that ellagic acid helps prevent and reduce certain cancers.[11] Scientists in

France have also studied ellagic acid's effect on mice with lung tumors—tumors that had been induced by carcinogens. These scientists found that ellagic acid, injected through the chest cavity or consumed, decreased the number of carcinogen-caused tumors.[42] And other research by Dr. R. L. Chang and colleagues at the Roche Research Center, the Memorial Sloan Kettering Cancer Center and the National Institutes of Health showed that treating mice with ellagic acid shortly before an injection of various carcinogens caused a 44 percent to 75 percent reduction in the number of lung tumors the mice developed.[43] In another study, Canadian researchers found that ellagic acid reduced lung-tumor development in mice by 54 percent.[44]

Certainly, animal studies don't always translate well to human subjects, but in the case of ellagic acid, research indicates that this phenolic does produce similar results in both animals and people. When you really think about it, this should not be surprising, because both humans and mice have about 30,000 genes, and only about 300 genes are unique to either species. In fact, scientists have recently found that "90 percent of genes associated with disease are identical in humans and mice."[45] Nonetheless, research into ellagic acid's protective effect on human tissues is described throughout this chapter as well.

First, ellagic acid has exhibited its anticancerous effects in esophageal tissues. For instance, the aforementioned Dr. Stoner, working with Dr. Swampa Mandal at the Medical College of Ohio, demonstrated how ellagic acid inhibited cancer in esophageal tissue by limiting DNA damage. Ellagic acid apparently inhibited the chemical capabilities of a carcinogen that causes DNA damage. And in the end, the ellagic acid reduced the development of esophageal lesions/tumors by between 21 percent and 50 percent.[46] In other research, Dr. Joseph C. Siglin at the Medical College of Ohio and his colleagues, including Dr. Stoner, found that ellagic acid effectively inhibited tumor formation in rats' esophagi when the acid was administered before, during, and after the administration of a carcinogen.[47] Dr. Elaine M. Daniel of the Medical College of Ohio and Dr. Stoner later demonstrated that ellagic acid could reduce the formation of carcinogen-induced esophageal tumors by 60 percent in rats.[48] And additional research by Dr. Mandal and others has shown that ellagic acid helps prevent DNA damage in human trachea and bronchial tissues.[49]

Ellagic acid has also been shown to be effective in cancerous liver tissues. For example, a team led by Dr. Takuji Tanaka of Japan's Gifu University School of Medicine investigated ellagic acid's effect on the formation of liver cancer in male rats. Rats were fed a diet containing ellagic acid before, during, and after the administration of a carcinogen. The result? The ellagic acid reduced the number of damaged cells and the incidence of tumors.[50] Additionally, in India during 2002, Dr. K. I. Priyadarsini and others showed that ellagic acid inhibits gamma-radiation-induced oxidation of fat in rats' liver cells.[51]

Other human tissues have also benefited from ellagic acid's anticancer properties. In Japan, Dr. Tanaka's team found that ellagic acid inhibits the formation of tumors and cancer in the tongue.[52] Also, teams led by Dr. Hasan Mukhtar at Case Western University and by Dr. H. U. Gali at Kansas State University separately found that ellagic acid protects against chemical-induced skin cancer.[53,54,55] Other research shows that ellagic acid inhibits certain carcinogen-induced chemical reactions, which can lead to cancers of the bladder,[56] of the brain's pineal gland,[57,58] of the pancreas,[59] of the prostate,[60] and of the colon.[61]

Ellagic acid's antioxidant properties help keep normal cells from becoming abnormal or cancerous cells.[62] By late 1990, researchers already had shown that use of ellagic acid reduces the cancer causing ability of several deadly carcinogenic chemicals; the list of carcinogens that ellagic acid has been found to inhibit has to continued to expand ever since.[42,43,46,49,50,53,54,63–66]

In addition, Drs. David Barch, Phillip M. Iannaccone, and Colleen C. Fox have demonstrated that a deficiency in dietary zinc increases the activities of certain carcinogens, and that ellagic acid can inhibit those same activities. And Drs. David Barch, and Lynn Rundhaugen have also demonstrated that consuming ellagic acid activates a number of cellular enzymes that detoxify carcinogens. Beyond that, these researchers found that ellagic acid also acts as a scavenger to bind and inactivate cancer-causing chemicals.[67,68,69]

All of these anticancerous benefits are welcome news. But of special concern to women and their loved ones are the constant threats of breast and cervical cancers. Thankfully, ellagic acid, as found in Georgian pomegranate, has been shown to help prevent the formation of breast and cervical cancer cells, and to inhibit and attack existing cancer cells in the cervix. We'll explore both of these specific cancers in detail.

BREAST CANCER

Breast cancer is second only to skin cancer as the most common form of cancer among women in the United States. The incidence of this disease has been rising for the past two decades, although researchers feel that much of the increase is associated with increased and improved screenings and detection. These improvements, along with better treatments, likely led to the significant decrease in breast cancer deaths between 1992 and 1996. Nonetheless, about 40,600 American women died from breast cancer during 2001.[70] And during 2002, an estimated 203,500 new cases of invasive breast cancer, plus an estimated 54,300 cases of in situ breast cancer, were diagnosed.[71,72] If current rates stay constant, the National Cancer Institute estimates that one in eight women will develop breast cancer sometime during their lives.[73]

The American Cancer Society lists several factors that can increase a woman's risk of developing breast cancer. These factors include:

- Advancing age
- Inheriting either of two mutated genes
- Having a family history of breast cancer
- Having a personal history of breast cancer
- Being Caucasian (i.e., "white")
- Having prior abnormal breast biopsies
- Being exposed to chest radiation as a child or young woman
- Experiencing the onset of menstruation before age twelve
- Experiencing the onset of menopause after age fifty

Table 13. Chances of being diagnosed with breast cancer by age groups

Age 30 to age 40	1 out of 252
Age 40 to age 50	1 out of 68
Age 50 to age 60	1 out of 35
Age 60 to age 70	1 out of 28
Age 70 to age 80	1 out of 27
Lifetime	1 out of 8

Source: National Cancer Institute. 2002.[73]

- Using birth-control pills within the last ten years
- Using hormone-replacement therapy
- Consuming alcoholic beverages
- Being overweight
- Lacking exercise[74]

Previously cited studies have described ellagic acid's ability to prevent, inhibit, reduce the number of, and even destroy cancer cells. In addition, research by Dr. Wendy A. Smith and her colleagues at the University of Kentucky's Graduate Center for Toxicology also shows that ellagic acid specifically helps prevent the earliest chemical reactions that can lead to the development of breast cancer.[75-78] To understand her team's findings, though, we first need a little background on one toxic chemical.

Dibenzopyrene (DBP) is a potentially deadly environmental chemical found in cigarette smoke, diesel exhaust, and other products of combustion. Rodent research has shown it is one of the most potent known mammary carcinogens. Therefore, it often is used in laboratories to create cancers in otherwise healthy cells and to allow these cancer-infected cells to be studied. Like other carcinogens, DBP metabolizes with enzymes to produce specific carcinogenic chemicals, which bind to DNA and corrupt it. When this damage goes unrepaired or misrepaired, the DNA produces mutant cells, which may become cancerous and proliferate.[79]

The good news is that Dr. Smith's team found that ellagic acid reduced the binding of DBP carcinogenic chemicals to breast cells' DNA by 45 percent, thereby reducing carcinogen bioactivation by 45 percent.

However, DBP can also bind directly to DNA without first metabolizing with enzymes to create carcinogenic chemicals. Fortunately, in another study in 1998, Dr. Smith's team looked at six cancer-preventive agents and found that ellagic acid was the only one that could inhibit DBP from binding directly to DNA in the absence of microsomal enzymes. The ellagic acid reduced the amount of direct DPB-to-DNA binding by 64 percent, thereby reducing carcinogen bioactivation by 64 percent.[75-78]

In other research, Dr. N. D. Kim of South Korea's Pusan National University led a team of scientists from the United States, Canada, Great Britain, and Israel in studying the anti-cancer effects of pomegranate phenolics extracted from pomegranate seeds and juice. In 2002, the researchers reported that pomegranate seed oil phenolics reduced the proliferation of breast cancer cells by 90 percent and reduced metastasizing (the spread of the cancer cells) by 75 percent. Then, in a test on another line of breast cancer cells, pomegranate seed oil phenolics caused the death of 54 percent of the cancer cells. And in yet another test, in which the doctors used a deadly carcinogen to induce cancer in rodent breast tissue, the pomegranate juice phenolics reduced the formation of cancerous lesions by 47 percent.[80]

CERVICAL CANCER

The American Cancer Society estimates that about 12,200 new cases of invasive cervical cancer were diagnosed in the United States during 2003. Also during 2003, about 4,100 women died from the disease. During the same period, about 48,800 additional women became victims of noninvasive cervical cancers.[81]

Human papillomaviruses are one of the primary risk factors for cervical cancer.[82] These papillomaviruses are viruses that can cause warts. Some are sexually transmitted and cause wart-like growths on the genitals. And although human papillomaviruses are best known as precursors to cervical cancer, they have also been associated with cancers of the skin, mouth, throat, tonsils, esophagus, stomach, rectum, anus, vulva, vagina, penis, and scrotum. [83-88]

Because human papilloma viruses are spread mainly through sexual contact, the risk of developing them increases with the number of sexual partners. Perhaps not surprising, then, is the fact that human papilloma virus infection is more common in younger age groups, particularly in women in their late teens and twenties. Women who become sexually active at a young age, who have multiple sexual partners, and whose sexual partners have other partners are at increased risk—though nonsexual transmission is also possible.[89]

Between 50 and 75 percent of sexually active men and women will be infected with genital human papillomavirus (HPV) at some point in their lives, and about 5.5 million Americans acquire new human papillomavirus infections each year.[89] In addition, the National Cancer Institute estimates that more than 6 million American women currently have chronic human papillomavirus infections.[90] A 2001 study revealed that 73 percent of women with low-grade squamous intraepithelial lesions and 89 percent of women with high-grade squamous intraepithelial lesions tested positive for human papillomaviruses infections. These women have the greatest risk of developing cervical cancer at some point in their lives. And of women who were already suffering from cervical cancer, 88 percent tested positive for human papillomaviruses.[91] However, results of wider epidemiological studies, and different and more sensitive methods of testing, are now indicating that human papilloma virus infection may be responsible for initiating up to 99 percent of all cervical cancer cases worldwide.[92,93,94]

More than 80 types of human papillomaviruses have been

identified. About 30 types infect the cervix, and 19 types are associated with cervical cancer.[91,93,94] These latter 19 types are called carcinogenic human papillomaviruses, and they are known by numbers: types 16, 18, 26, 31, 33, 35, 39, 45, 51, 52, 53, 56, 58, 59, 66, 67, 68, 73, and 82.[90,91,94,95,96] It is not uncommon for a person infected with human papillomavirus to be infected with two or more types of the virus simultaneously.[84,96]

"The evidence implicating papillomavirus as an etiologic agent of cervical cancer has come from a variety of observational laboratory studies," according to Dr. William C. Reeves and his colleagues at the Gorgas Memorial Laboratory. "Genital papillomaviruses induce dysplastic lesions. Most invasive cervical cancers contain papillomavirus DNA, as do cell lines derived from cervical cancers. Viral DNA appears to be integrated into cellular DNA, and integration involves highly conserved, transcriptionally active regions of the viral DNA. It also is clear from the epidemiological evidence that cervical cancer has a multifactorial etiology, which also can involve cofactors such as pregnancy, smoking, use of hormonal contraceptives, and diet."[97]

The good news is that Dr. B. A. Narayanan and her colleagues at the Hollings Cancer Center of the Medical University of South Carolina have found that ellagic acid can make a difference in fighting cervical cancer. Narayanan and her team found that ellagic acid stopped cancer cell mutation within forty-eight hours, inhibited overall cell growth, and induced cervical cancer cells' death after seventy-two hours of treatment. The phenolic appeared to activate a certain protein, and this activation "suggests a role for ellagic acid in cell-cycle regulation of cancer cells," according to the researchers.[98]

The cancer cell line on which this ellagic acid study was performed was called CaSki. This cell line carries human papillomavirus type 16,[98] and epidemiological studies have indicated that human papillomavirus type 16 is the most commonly found and the most dangerous of all carcinogenic human papillomaviruses.[87,88,91,94,95] Therefore, ellagic acid's ability to inhibit cancer formation in this cell line is particularly significant.

TOBACCO-RELATED CANCERS

Tobacco is responsible for nearly one in five deaths in the United States, whether it comes in the form of cigarettes, cigars, pipe tobacco, or snuff. Approximately half of all people who smoke cigarettes, and continue to smoke, will die from smoking-related diseases—primarily lung cancer—and half of those people will die during middle age, or between the ages of thirty-five and sixty-nine. Lung cancer, the most common tobacco-related cancer, produces no noticeable symptoms in its early stages, and therefore, in 85 percent of all people who develop it, the cancer spreads before it is detected. Overall, this cancer is so deadly that the one-year survival rate of lung cancer sufferers is only 41 percent, and the five-year survival rate is only 15 percent.

Of course, people who quit smoking dramatically reduce their chances of developing lung cancer, and the younger they are when they quit smoking, the better the prognosis. Nevertheless, because of the damage smoking does to cells, ex-smokers maintain a 15 percent higher than normal risk of developing lung cancer sometime during their lives. For many people, far too much damage is done before the smoking addiction is finally broken. This explains why 50 percent of all lung cancers are diagnosed in the 23 percent of American adults who are former smokers. Smoking is also associated with cancers of the mouth, pharynx, larynx, esophagus, pancreas, uterus, cervix, kidney, and bladder.

People who have never smoked are also at risk for developing tobacco-related cancers. Secondhand smoke has been shown to contain more than 4,000 chemicals, 40 of which are known or suspected carcinogens. And long-term snuff users are nearly 50 times more likely than nonusers to develop cancers of the cheek and gums.[18,99,100,101] Thus, current tobacco users, former tobacco users, and nonsmokers all need to protect themselves from the carcinogenic chemicals and chemical by-products of tobacco.[102,103]

Fortunately, research shows that ellagic acid helps protect human cells against some of the carcinogens that occur in tobacco smoke. For example, ellagic acid has been shown to fight one of the most potent tobacco carcinogens, NNK. Drs. R. W. Teel and A. Castonguay of California's Loma Linda University School of Medicine tested various phenolics, including ellagic acid, to see if they could reduce the occurrence of genetic mutations caused by the chemical NNK. These genetic mutations lead to cancer. In the end, the researchers found that ellagic acid reduced the occurrence of mutations by 67 percent.[104]

And in a later study, ellagic acid again proved effective against tobacco-related carcinogens—as did phenolics in two of the other plants discussed in this book. Swedish researchers examined fifteen compounds that had all been suggested as inhibitors of the mutagen-creating properties of a cigarette smoke by-product and an extract of oral Swedish moist snuff. The compounds included ellagic acid (found in abundance in Georgian pomegranate), chlorogenic acid (found in abundance in Caucasian blueberry leaves and in *Rhododendron caucasicum*), and (+)-catechin hydrate, which is also found in *Rhododendron caucasicum*. In the final analysis, the test results indicated that ellagic acid almost completely inhibited the mutagen-producing capability of cigarette smoke condensate and Swedish moist snuff. Chlorogenic acid also strongly inhibited the mutagen-producing capability of both substances, and (+)–catechin reduced the mutagen-producing capability of Swedish moist snuff.[105]

MORE CANCER-RELATED PROTECTION

Research on ellagic acid, which occurs in Georgian pomegranates in extremely high amounts, provides us with even more examples of this phenolic's cancer-fighting properties. These include another example of protecting the lungs from the formation of tumors, and reducing the severity of alcohol-related stomach lesions—lesions that increase people's risk of developing gastrointestinal cancers. Research also reveals that Georgian pomegranate juice contains far more powerful free radical neutralizers than green tea.

Indian researchers studied ellagic acid's potential against the formation of lung tumors in mice. They found that the phenolic reduced the rate of tumor formation to 20 percent of normal. In addition, they found that quercetin, a flavonoid in both *Rhododendron caucasicum* and Caucasian blueberry leaves, also produced good results by reducing the rate of tumor formation to 44.4 percent of normal. And both ellagic acid and quercetin suppressed tumor development mainly by acting at the formation phase of the cancer.[106]

Ellagic acid also proved effective against one factor that can lead to the development of gastrointestinal cancers: the gastric lesions that come with the frequent consumption of alcoholic beverages.[107,108] Researchers at Japan's Kyoto Pharmaceutical University found that ellagic acid could reduce the severity of the stomach lesions caused by whiskey and ethanol alcohol consumption. The scientists believe ellagic acid's protective action comes from the nutrient's antioxidant and anti-inflammatory activities.[109,110]

Finally, Dr. Can-Lan Sun and his colleagues at the University of Southern California have found that people who drink green tea have a 50 percent lower risk of developing gastric and esophageal cancers, thanks to the antioxidant activity of the green tea's phenolics.[111,112] But pomegranate juice phenolics have been shown to possess three times the antioxidant activity of green tea (and of red wine).[113] Thus, with its even more potent phenolic composition, which includes ellagic acid, Georgian pomegranate juice should be even more effective against certain cancers.

Additional Health Solutions

As one of the greatest plant sources of ellagic acid, the Georgian pomegranate is destined to become well known in preventing and treating cancer. However, some of the same antioxidant properties that help the pomegranate inhibit the onset and spread of cancers are also effective against other deleterious health conditions, including high blood pressure, arterial and heart inflammation, and atherosclerosis. In addition, the pomegranate can help protect the liver and kidneys from free radical damage, fight bacteria, and promote the activity of other antioxidants.

ATHEROSCLEROSIS

As described in Chapter 4, research now shows that LDLs (bad cholesterol) modified by oxidation (or turned into free radicals by other free radicals or toxins) are absorbed by arterial macrophage cells at an advanced rate, which thereby quickens the formation of arterial plaque.[114,115] And as also previously described, HDLs (good cholesterol) help control LDL levels by scavenging LDLs from the blood vessel walls and transporting them back to the liver for further processing and disposal. However, as noted, HDL molecules can also be converted into dangerous free radicals through oxidation.[116-119]

Fortunately, one way pomegranate juice appears to help prevent arterial plaque from forming is by enhancing the activity of a free-radical-destroying enzyme called paraoxonase.

Professor Michael Aviram, D.Sc., head of the Lipid Research Laboratory at Technion Israel Institute of Technology, has revealed that the enzyme paraoxonase, which binds to HDLs, appears to protect both HDLs and LDLs from oxidation. Specifically, paraoxonase can decompose certain free-radical-producing toxins. However, paraoxonase can also be inactivated by free radicals, including oxidized LDLs and HDLs. Thus, any kind of interventions that could preserve or enhance paraoxonase activity might help fight atherosclerosis and forestall the onset and progression of coronary heart disease.[120-123]

Well, pioneering research by Dr. Michael Aviram and colleagues has shown that pomegranate can provide just the right kind of intervention. Dr. Aviram's team demonstrated that supplementing the body with pomegranate increased the activity of the paraoxonase enzyme.[124]

Subsequent research by Dr. Marielle Kaplan and colleagues at Technion and other Israeli research centers also showed that pomegranate juice significantly increased paraoxonase activity in mice. Furthermore, Dr. Kaplan's team found that by administering pomegranate juice, they could reduce macrophage cells' absorption of oxidized LDLs by 31 percent and increase the release of cholesterol from macrophage cells by 39 percent.[125]

In other research, Dr. Michael Aviram's team has found that pomegranate juice prevents the buildup of plaque in mice arteries, and that it inhibits damaging changes in mice that already have plaque in their arteries. The researchers found they could use pomegranate juice to reduce LDL oxidation by up to 90 percent in mice that were susceptible to heart disease. Furthermore, they found that when the mice at risk for heart disease drank pomegranate juice for eleven weeks, the juice reduced the size of the atherosclerotic lesions in the mice's arteries by 44 percent. The juice also reduced the mice's total number of foam cells, which are associated with heart disease.[124]

But beyond studies of mice, science has also shown pomegranate's effectiveness against atherosclerosis in humans. For example, Dr. Aviram's team also analyzed the effect of pomegranate juice consumption on the processes that lead to atherosclerosis in healthy, male volunteers. These effects were assessed after the subjects drank only two to three ounces of pomegranate juice daily for two weeks. In the end, the juice decreased LDLs' susceptibility to macrophage absorption and retention, and it increased paraoxonase activity by 18 percent.[124]

It is interesting to note that this human study also compared the effects of pomegranate juice to those of pomegranate peel, and that extract made from the peel demonstrated higher antioxidant activity. The major phenolic in pomegranate peel is ellagic acid.[124] Also interesting is a comment Dr. Aviram made after completing his studies. He said he chose pomegranates for his research because the fruit had long been used in folk medicines to treat infections and disease. He suspected that some of its medicinal value could be due to antioxidants.[126]

HIGH BLOOD PRESSURE

Approximately 50 million Americans suffer from high blood pressure, and an additional 45 million are at risk of developing it based upon blood-pressure readings high enough to be categorized as prehypertension.[127] Of the first 50 million, only 70 percent are aware of their condition, only 59 percent are being treated for it, and only 34 percent have the condition under control. Thus, it is no surprise that during 1999 high blood pressure caused 14,308 U.S. deaths and led to 32 million visits to doctor's offices.[128]

High blood pressure is, in fact, the most frequently diagnosed adverse health condition.[129] It can be both a cause and an effect of atherosclerosis.[130-133] And besides increasing the risk of heart attacks, strokes, congestive heart failure, and dementia, it can cause kidney failure and eye damage.[134]

One class of drugs used to treat patients with high blood pressure contains substances called angiotensin-converting enzyme inhibitors, or ACE inhibitors. Angiotensin-converting enzyme is a chemical that causes the arteries to constrict and tighten, thus adding to the heart's workload and increasing

Table 14. Blood Pressure Levels

Blood Pressure	Systolic (Top number)	Diastolic (Bottom number)
Normal	Less than 120	Less than 80
Prehypertension	120 to 139	80 to 90
Hypertension	140 or higher	90 or higher

Source: Chobanian et al., 2003.[127]

blood pressure. ACE inhibitors, on the other hand, relax the blood vessels and reduce blood pressure. Now, research has shown that reducing ACE activity, even without reducing blood pressure, slows the progress of atherosclerosis.[135,136,137]

Fortunately, pomegranate juice has been shown to reduce ACE activity. For example, Israeli Drs. Michael Aviram and Leslie Dornfeld studied the effect of pomegranate juice consumption on patients with high blood pressure. They found that consuming 50 milliliters of pomegranate juice per day for two weeks resulted in a 5 percent reduction in systolic blood pressure and a 36 percent reduction in ACE activity.[137]

ARTERIAL AND HEART INFLAMMATION

When arteries have been injured by free radicals, bacterial and/or viral infections, hypertension, or any stage of atherosclerotic plaque buildup, they become subject to further damage and narrowing as a result of inflammation caused by two enzymes, cyclooxygenase and lipoxygenase. These two enzymes turn fatty acids into inflammation-producing hormones. These enzymes are active in any injured area of the body. Research has shown that inhibiting the cyclooxygenase and lipoxygenase enzymes mitigates artery damage while further limiting symptoms of atherosclerosis.[138] Now, research has shown the pomegranate to be an effective cyclooxygenase and lipoxygenase inhibitor.

Dr. Shay Schubert and his colleagues at Technion Israel Institute of Technology investigated the pomegranate's antioxidant properties and its ability to inhibit cyclooxygenase and lipoxygenase. They looked specifically at cyclooxygenase from sheep and lipoxygenase from soybeans because these enzymes react similarly to their human counterparts. Overall, the team found that flavonoids extracted from pomegranate juice reduced the activity of soybean lipoxygenase by between 21 percent and 30 percent. Furthermore, flavonoids extracted from pomegranate seed oil reduced the inflammatory activity of sheep cyclooxygenase by between 31 percent and 44 percent, and reduced soybean lipoxygenase activity by between 69 percent and 81 percent. All of the studied flavonoids showed strong antioxidant activity.[139] Interestingly, like Dr. Aviram, Dr. Schubert also said he chose to use pomegranates for his study because of the fruit's historical use in folk medicines and because he suspected that some of the pomegranate's medicinal value could be due to antioxidants.[140]

In addition to fighting arterial inflammation, pomegranate's powerful ellagic acid also has been proven effective against inflammation in the heart. This power was demonstrated by Dr. L. V. Iakovleva and colleagues at the Ukrainian Pharmaceutical Academy who administered ellagic acid to rats suffering from myocarditis, or inflammation of the heart's muscular walls. In the end, Dr. Iakovleva's team found that ellagic acid reversed disturbed myocardial functions, thus preventing long-term damage from inflammation.[141]

KIDNEY AND LIVER PROTECTION

Georgian pomegranate's ellagic acid has also been shown to help protect the body from several additional potential adverse conditions. In particular, it can protect the kidneys and liver from nickel damage and damage from carbon tetrachloride.

Nickel can be a major environmental pollutant—deadly when ingested or inhaled in large amounts. Nickel is known to cause breaks in the chromosomes that carry our genetic material, and it causes pathological alterations to the kidneys, liver, and blood serum.[142,143] Fortunately, as noted, ellagic acid can help prevent nickel damage.

For example, scientists in the Department of Medical Elementology and Toxicology at India's Hamdard University poisoned rats with nickel to create abnormal blood chemistries indicative of kidney and liver malfunction. Then they administered ellagic acid and observed the results. As it turned out, the ellagic acid caused the nickel to be excreted from cells and tissues, thus greatly reducing nickel-induced toxicity. The reduction in toxicity was clear when levels of seven key chemical indicators improved following ellagic acid administration. Of these results, team leader Hamdard's Dr. Ahmed said, "Our data suggests that ellagic acid acts as an effective chelating agent in suppressing nickel-induced renal [kidney] and hepatic [liver] biochemical alterations. . . . Ellagic acid maintains cell membrane integrity."[142]

Another compound, this one a manufactured substance called carbon tetrachloride, causes severe liver toxicity, and chronic exposure to it can produce fibrosis (excess fibrous connective tissue) in the liver.[144,145] Fortunately, ellagic acid has also proven effective against this compound. In fact, researchers at India's Amala Cancer Research Centre found that administering ellagic acid to animals that had been exposed to carbon tetrachloride significantly reduced danger-ously elevated levels of enzymes, liver hydroxy proline, and lipid peroxide—and it rectified liver health.[144]

PROTECTION AGAINST BACTERIAL INFECTION

Pomegranate ellagic acid extract has also proven effective against various bacteria. For example, it can inhibit *Pseudomonas aeruginosa*, dysentery bacteria, and typhoid bac-teria. And when compared with eleven other plant extracts used in traditional Mexican medicine to cure infectious *Staphylococcus aureus, E. coli (Escherichia coli), Pseudomonas aeruginosa,* and *Candida albicans,* the pomegranate extract revealed the strongest anti-microbal activity against the tested microorganisms.[11] In addition, scientists at the University of Iowa have demonstrated that ellagic acid inhibits certain oral pathogens, including *Porphyromonas gingivalis* and *Prevotella intermedia.*[146]

GLUTATHIONE

Finally, Georgian pomegranate's ellagic acid has been shown to promote the activity of other antioxidants, particularly one called glutathione.

Glutathione is a powerful antioxidant produced by the cells and found in almost every cell of the human body. It protects and helps regulate all human systems,[147] and its importance is evidenced by its mention in more than 50,000 published scientific studies.[148] In general, high levels of glutathione are associated with good health, and low levels of glutathione are associated with poor health—including chronic and deadly diseases.[147]

As reported in the journal *Food and Chemical Toxicology,* ellagic acid, as found in Georgian pomegranate, has been shown to significantly increase the availability of glutathione.[106] In addition, other special antioxidants found in *Rhododendron caucasicum,* Caucasian blueberry leaves, and *Rhodiola rosea* (which will be discussed in the next chapter) have also been shown to increase the availability of glutathione and thus help ensure the body's overall good health.[149]

In the end, ellagic acid's antioxidant-enhancing power and other disease-fighting properties are what make Georgian pomegranate such an important plant. Truly, along with the other plants mentioned in this book, it can help maintain good health, prevent disease, and promote longevity in unique ways.

Choosing a Pomegranate/Ellagic Acid Extract

News of ellagic acid's tremendous anticancer properties is spreading rapidly around the world. More and more people are seeking plant extracts which contain this powerful phenolic antioxidant in order to protect and maintain their health. However, before people make a decision about an ellagic acid product, there are a few things they should know about percentages of ellagic acid and about good extract standards.

ELLAGIC ACID PERCENTAGE

The first thing to realize is that ellagic acid is ellagic acid, and even a slight variation in the ellagic acid's molecular structure would make the substance into something completely different. In other words, all true ellagic acid is chemically identical. The difference in ellagic acid products, then, is the plant material in which ellagic acid is contained, as well as the fillers that are sometimes added by encapsulators.

When you purchase an ellagic acid product, it contains a standard amount of phenolics including ellagic acid. This standard is expressed as a percentage of the product's total source plant material. The balance of the capsule contains that plant material, which could be bayberries, blackberries, blueberries, cranberries, feijoa, grapes, pecans, pineapple, pomegranate, raspberries, walnuts, or strawberries, and sometimes fillers. Each of the plant substances provides its own unique and beneficial phytochemical complexes, which include ellagic acid. Therefore, it is really up to you to decide which phytochemical complexes you desire to consume.

One of the many good things about Georgian pomegranate ellagic acid extract is that it is standardized to 40 percent ellagic acid. This means that 40 percent of Georgian pomegranate raw material is composed of ellagic acid. Since the extract's total polyphenolic content is 70 percent, this means that nearly half the phenolics in Georgian pomegranate ellagic acid extract are phenolics other than ellagic acid.[11,150]

In contrast, many ellagic acid products currently available in the United States are composed of raspberry ellagic acid extract. Raspberries provide an abundance of beneficial phytonutrients, including ellagic acid. However, raspberries naturally consist of 100 times less ellagic acid per gram than pomegranate (0.01% vs. 1%) and, because of this, it is cost prohibitive to produce a raspberry ellagic acid extract that exceeds 2% of the raspberry plant material in a product. Therefore, as most often is the case, 100 milligrams of a raspberry ellagic acid extract product would provide a maximum of 2 milligrams of ellagic acid, whereas 100 milligrams of a pomegranate ellagic acid extract product would provide 40 milligrams of ellagic acid.[151]

Undoubtedly, someone will eventually add extra ellagic acid to raspberry ellagic acid products. But because raspberries are composed of only 0.01 percent ellagic acid, the additional ellagic acid probably will have to come from another source. If this occurs, the consumer should make sure that the ellagic acid used to boost the raspberry ellagic acid product is a natural, plant-derived ellagic acid rather than a synthetic analog, such as the Chinese and others have been attempting to develop.[151] After all, most Americans are careful to purchase only natural vitamin E rather than synthetic vitamin E, and the same care should be taken when purchasing ellagic acid products.

OTHER KEY CONSIDERATIONS

As with the other plant extracts previously discussed, when choosing an ellagic acid product, consumers should also consider whether herbicides, pesticides, or toxic organic solvents were used in cultivating or extracting the product.

As has been noted, when herbicides or pesticides are used in cultivation, their residues often remain on the plant material contained in the product capsules.[152,153] These residues can produce powerful free radicals. However, since Georgian pomegranate is wild crafted, which means it grows in the wild and is harvested from herbicide- and pesticide-free land, consumers can be assured that they are getting a truly herbicide-free and pesticide-free product.

Additionally, and as has been mentioned, almost all other plant-based nutritional substances are extracted using toxic organic solvents. When this happens, the solvents' residues remain on the plant material contained in the product capsules, and again, these residues produce free radicals. In contrast, Georgian pomegranate ellagic acid extract, like the other extracts described in this book, is extracted without the use of toxic organic solvents.

Based on the aforementioned, and for reasons of both effectiveness and value, consumers should be sure that any ellagic acid product they purchase, regardless of the plant source, conforms to the following specifications:

• The extract is composed of at least 40 percent ellagic acid.

- The plants from which it was extracted were cultivated without the use of herbicides or pesticides.
- Its plant material was extracted and processed without the use of toxic solvents.

Ancient Wisdom, Modern Science

Georgians and other ancient peoples have used the pomegranate to protect their health for thousands of years. Now, modern science is catching on. During the last few decades, biochemical, pharmacological, and clinical studies have been performed at leading scientific research centers which prove the effectiveness of pomegranate and its key constituent, ellagic acid. Clearly, pomegranate is one of the world's greatest known sources of ellagic acid—a powerful antioxidant and anticancer phytochemical that has been described in more than five hundred studies published during the last thirty-seven years. Studies have revealed pomegranate's tremendous effectiveness at slowing the onset and progression of cancer and atherosclerosis, and at lowering high blood pressure, inhibiting dangerous inflammatory processes, and protecting the kidneys and liver from environmental pollutants. An ancient plant that provides unique and powerful free radical neutralizing activity, pomegranate is destined to hold a venerable place in preventive medicine, along with the other three plants described here.

Next, in the book's final chapter, we'll explore the benefits of *Rhodiola rosea*, the last of four of the most important plants used by long-living Georgians.

CHAPTER 6

Rhodiola Rosea

Rhodiola rosea, Siberia's golden root, is a green leafy plant with yellow flowers which, at maturity, reaches a height of about two and a half feet. *Rhodiola rosea* is indigenous to the arctic regions of Europe, Eurasia, and Siberian Asia, where it grows at high altitudes in mountainous terrains. The plant also has been found growing on the Altai Mountains of southern Siberia and, to a far lesser extent, on the Caucasian Mountains on the republic of Georgia's northern border. And while the leaves of *Rhodiola rosea* are used for some treatments and in various foods, it is the gold-colored root of the plant which has been most effectively utilized in medicine for over 2,000 years.[1,2,3]

Though not indigenous to Georgia, *Rhodiola rosea* has been consumed by several generations of many long-living Georgians.[1] Today, with twinkles in their eyes, Georgian centenarians still toast the plant, saying, "Whoever drinks *Rhodiola rosea* tea will live more than 100 years."[1,3]

Research confirms *Rhodiola rosea*'s medicinal powers, and virtually anyone who consumes *Rhodiola rosea* will notice an impressive improvement in mental and physical performance. It is because of *Rhodiola rosea*'s obvious benefits, as well as its other medicinal properties, that *Rhodiola rosea* was a closely held performance secret of Soviet athletes and cosmonauts.[1]

Medicinal History of Rhodiola

The Greek physician Dioscorides noted *Rhodiola rosea*'s medicinal applications in about the year 77 A.D. in his *De Materia Medica*, where he referred to the plant as Rodia riza. Later, in the mid-1700s, Carl von Linné, who has been called the father of taxonomy, gave the plant its botanical and

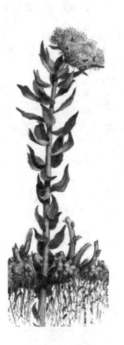

Rhodiola rosea

species names, *Rhodiola rosea L.*[4] Now, however, research indicates that *Rhodiola rosea* has been used by certain Siberians to protect health and treat specific illnesses since before the time of Christ.[1,4]

The plant has been a precious, cherished commodity for so many hundreds of years because of its unique medicinal properties. In fact, for several centuries, foreign emperors sent expeditions (sometimes illegally) into Siberia to obtain *Rhodiola rosea* from the high and wild places where it still grows.[2,4] And for nearly a thousand years, Siberian traders secreted the plant down ancient trails, south to the Caucasian Mountains. There, the Georgians would trade their wonderful wines, citrus fruits, garlic, and money for *Rhodiola rosea's* precious golden roots.[1]

This lust for Siberia's botanical treasures, including *Rhodiola rosea* and Siberian ginseng, continues today, as documented in a recent article in Siberia's *Vladivostok Daily* newspaper:

March 23, 2001
The Vladivostok Daily

"As the hunting and harvesting of wild plants started, border guards of Russia and China have posted additional patrols to curb rising numbers of Chinese residents crossing over into the Russian taiga, the Federal Border Guard Service reported on Monday.

"A press release from the service said that the Chinese citizens penetrate as far as four kilometers into Russian territory to pick edible and medicinal species of plants. . . . They often operate in organized groups.

"Border guards in Primorye detained 13 such perpetrators last week. . . .

"According to an agreement reached at a joint meeting last month, Russia has formed three extra patrols in Primorye, while China has posted four of them."[5]

In Siberian folk medicine, *Rhodiola rosea* was primarily used to increase physical endurance and work productivity, to reduce depression and fatigue, to provide resistance to high-altitude sickness, and to provide resistance to and treatment for colds and flu during frigid Siberian winters and chilly, damp springs. In addition, it was used to treat anemia, impotence, infections, vaginal discharges, gastrointestinal disorders, headaches, and hysteria. Its roots were even given to couples prior to marriage to assist in the birth of healthy children.[1,4]

Research indicates that *Rhodiola rosea* has long been used by certain Siberians to protect health and treat specific illnesses. News of *Rhodiola rosea*'s efficacies was passed down from elders through more than one hundred generations spanning over two thousand years. From 1979 to 1989, one of the most precious gifts Siberian mothers could send to their sons serving for the Soviets in the Afghanistan War were roots of *Rhodiola rosea*—gifts sent to help their sons reduce stress, depression and fatigue, and to protect general health.[1,6]

Outside of Siberia, other cultures found different uses for the plant. Mongolian doctors prescribed *Rhodiola rosea* for tuberculosis and cancer.[2,7] In many cultures, including Georgia, the plant's roots were used to extend healthy longevity, increase physical endurance, and gain clarity and peace of mind.[1,2] Vikings used *Rhodiola rosea* to increase their physical strength,[8] and German scientists wrote of its use as a stimulant and anti-inflammatory, and of its effectiveness at treating pain, headache, scurvy, and hemorrhoids.[9]

Now, almost everything that past peoples understood about *Rhodiola rosea*'s health benefits has been validated by science. The research began in the 1700s and has continued through today. Between 1749 and 1961, *Rhodiola rosea*'s medicinal applications were described in the scientific literature of Estonia, France, Georgia, Germany, Greece, Iceland, Norway, Russia, the Soviet Union, and Sweden. Between 1961 and 1988, more than one hundred pharmacological and clinical studies were performed on *Rhodiola rosea* and published in scientific literature.[4] During the last fifteen years, at least thirty more pharmacological and clinical studies on the plant have been published, and seventeen of these very recent studies came during the last two and a half years alone.[10] *Rhodiola rosea* has also been the subject of a recent article in *Newsweek* magazine and a scientific monograph coauthored by researchers from Columbia University, New York Medical Center, and Las Palmas Technological Institute in Spain.[6,11]

Clearly, this plant has something special to offer everyone interested in protecting their health. But what makes it so effective medicinally? One reason may be that *Rhodiola rosea* is both an antioxidant and an adaptogen. In fact, while many plant species exhibit various antioxidant properties, *Rhodiola rosea* is one of only a handful of plants classified as an adaptogen—a substance that helps animals and humans adapt to the changes and stresses of life.

A Proven Adaptogen

While the desire to help the body adapt to stresses was generated by the pioneering stress research of Dr. Walter Cannon of Harvard and Dr. Hans Selye of the University of Montreal, it was Russian doctor Nicholi Lazarev who did the first research on adaptogens and coined the term "adaptogen," and it is Russian scientists who have been the leaders in adaptogen research.[12–16]

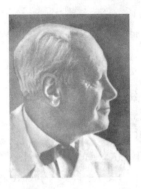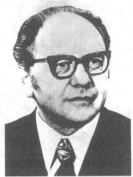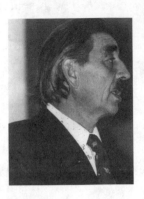

Israel I. Brekhman, Ph.D. (left), and Igor V. Dardymov, D.S. (right);
pioneers in the area of adaptogen research

In April 1969, Soviet pharmacologists Israel I. Brekhman and
Igor V. Dardymov published a landmark paper on adaptogens in
the *Annual Review of Pharmacology*.[17] The paper was titled "New
Substances of Plant Origin which Increase Nonspecific
Resistance," and even today, this work is the foundation for adaptogen research worldwide. In it, Drs. Brekhman and Dardymov
defined the criteria that any medicinal plant must meet to be
classified as an adaptogen. These criteria include the following:

- An adaptogen should be innocuous and cause minimal disorders in the physiological functions of an organism. In
  other words, it should not cause harm, nor should it lessen
  the performance of one system while improving the performance of another system.
- The action of an adaptogen should be nonspecific. In other
  words, it should increase resistance to a wide range of harmful physical, chemical, and biological factors.
- An adaptogen should possess normalizing action irrespec-
  tive of the direction of the previous pathological changes.

For example, if a pulse rate is too fast, it should slow it, and if a pulse rate is too slow, it should increase it.

Brekhman and Dardymov then investigated 189 medicinal plants to determine if they were adaptogens. In the end, only five met the requirements, one of which was *Rhodiola rosea*.[11,17]

Health Solutions

Because of its unique adaptogenic and antioxidant properties, *Rhodiola rosea* provides resistance to conditions that put stress on the human organism. It improves mental performance, including increasing short- and long-term memory; improves physical performance; and increases resistance to the harmful effects of radiation, toxins, cold, strenuous exercise, and too much or too little oxygen.[4] *Rhodiola rosea* also protects against free radical damage,[18] enhances DNA repair,[19] suppresses tumor growth,[11] helps reduce metastasizing of certain cancers,[20-24] lessens stress-induced damage to the heart,[25,26] promotes proper coronary flow following obstruction,[27] prevents certain arrhythmias,[27,28] and regenerates the liver,[1,22,29,30] among other benefits.

Many of these benefits will be discussed here, but we'll begin with the two effects that have made *Rhodiola rosea* the most famous: the successful prevention and treatment of depression and stress.[3,4,31]

DEPRESSION AND STRESS

Depression and stress often go hand in hand, which is why we'll discuss them concurrently. To begin, let's take a closer look at depression.

Depression. Depression strikes people of all social classes, races, and cultures and has been recognized as a health disorder for some 2,000 years.[32,33] These days, in any given year about 18.8 million American adults suffer from some sort of depressive illness.[34] Approximately 35 million to 40 million Americans living today will suffer major depressive episodes during their lives, and typically, the first episode will occur between the ages of 25 and 44. The incidence of depression will then increase with age. Regardless of age, depression affects women twice as often as men. The National Foundation for Depressive Illnesses estimates that the cost of lost productivity, replacement personnel, medical care, and loss of life due to depression totals between $15 billion and $35 billion per year in the United States.[35]

People who are depressed experience overwhelming inner sadness, which can manifest itself in a number of symptoms. These symptoms include guilt, shame, low self-esteem, negative thoughts and speech, a preoccupation with death or dying, reduced concentration, reduced productivity, antisocial behavior, weight changes, too much or too little sleep, and decreased interest in sex. In most cases, those who are depressed also suffer from energy loss and become less active; however, some become hyperactive.[32,36]

Research reveals that depression increases the risk of cardiovascular diseases,[37] including heart attack,[38] stroke,[39] and hypertension.[40] It also affects the heart rate after a heart attack,[41] and in fact, the depressed are three to four times more likely to die within six months of having a heart attack than are nondepressed heart-attack victims.[42] People suffering from depression also are at increased risk for developing Alzheimer's disease,[43] Parkinson's disease,[44] dementia,[45] seizures (in older adults),[46] osteoporosis,[47] early premenopause,[48] gastrointestinal disorders, and diabetes,[49] among other illnesses. Additionally, people who suffer from depression are three times less likely to comply with medical recommendations.[50] They and their families also have dramatically shorter life spans.[51]

Stress. Uncontrolled stress can lead to all types of maladies, including concomitant depression. As Drs. Zakir Ramazanov and Maria del Mar Bernal Suarez wrote in their book *New Secrets of Effective Natural Stress and Weight Management Using Rhodiola Rosea and Rhododendron Caucasicum,* "It is an unfortunate fact that about 80 percent of all illnesses can be tracked back to stress."[52] Furthermore, the organization Psych-Net Mental Health has estimated that 75 percent to 90 percent of all visits to primary care physicians are stress-related.[53] With percentages like these, it is no surprise that Vladimir Bernik, M.D., the author of *Stress: The Silent Killer,* has estimated that stress-related illnesses cost American businesses $50 billion to $300 billion per year in lost productivity.[54]

So what are some of the illnesses to which stress contributes? "Many studies have shown the deleterious effects that stress has on general immunity in the body," wrote Drs. Ramazanov and del Mar Bernal Suarez. "One study found that medical students showed a higher risk of getting mononucleosis during examination periods than during less stressful times. Children exposed to high levels of stress were shown to have lowered immunity in the lungs than children who were not stressed."[55] Additional findings reveal that stress causes more frequent herpes simplex Type 1 outbreaks and that stress increases susceptibility to the effects of Epstein-Barr virus infection.[56,57] Stress lessens the effectiveness of vaccines,[58] makes us more vulnerable to influenza,[59] and lengthens the time it takes for wounds to heal.[60,61] It also speeds the progression of cancer and infectious illnesses, including

AIDS,[62] and stress has been shown to decrease the activity of the immune system's natural killer cells, which inhibit viral replication and are a first line of defense against cancer.[63,64] Additionally, stress increases our pulse rate, blood pressure, and blood clotting, each of which increases the risk of heart attacks and strokes.[65,66] It makes gastrointestinal problems and asthma worse, and it intensifies pain[67] and reduces energy, enthusiasm, productivity, and concentration.[68] Finally, stress also has been shown to cause the production of inflammatory cytokines, which promote several aging illnesses, including cardiovascular disease, osteoporosis, arthritis, Type 2 diabetes, certain cancers, Alzheimer's disease, and periodontal disease.[69]

Harvard Medical School's renown professor of dermatology, T. B. Fitzpatrick, has described additional stress-related health disorders in his research. His studies show that stress, fatigue, and other emotional problems are responsible for 95 percent of wart outbreaks, 76 percent of hand eczema, 70 percent of atopic eczema, 15 percent of contact eczema, 68 percent of hives, and 55 percent of acne outbreaks. All of these conditions occur in as little as a few seconds or up to two days after an emotional trigger.[70,71]

Stress also can trigger neuroses[72,73,74] and other debilitating psychological disorders.[75] One of those disorders is asthenia, which is also a symptom of depression and several other conditions.[76,77,78] Asthenia is characterized by mental and physical fatigue, labored breathing, irritability, giddiness, sleep disturbances, chest pain, rapid pulse rate, anxiety, decline in work capacity, poor appetite, and headaches[79,80] It most often occurs in individuals exposed to stressful conditions, especially intense mental demands.

Stress can be caused by myriad external and internal stimuli, from exposure to cold or heat to having an unpleasant thought.[81,82] Interestingly, a single stimulus can cause a stress response that results in more than 1,400 known chemical reactions in the body.[83]

Often stress can be controlled and dissipated, but if it is not controlled, its intensity can increase. It is compounded by additional stress from the stress itself and by additional stimuli, including depression. The fact is that the damaging effects of uncontrolled stress are cumulative. Therefore, stress must be prevented, controlled, and dissipated in order to avoid the more serious problems it can bring.

Many of us are familiar with the famous Social Readjustment Rating Scale of the 1960s.[84] This test allowed readers to gauge their susceptibility to illness according to the stressful events they experienced. Point values were assigned to the stressful events people typically experienced during the preceding twelve-month period, and various point levels indicated susceptibility to illness. While this test seemed reasonable enough at the time, few researchers in the late 1960s could have imagined how dramatically the pace of life would accelerate during the next thirty-plus years. Many new conveniences have actually increased rather than decreased our responsibilities and work loads, and all of these must be handled in an environment of increased traffic of every form and increased social expectations. Today, it therefore seems reasonable that several additional stress points could be scored by every person living and working during this first decade of the twenty-first century. And new point totals would undoubtedly show that tens of millions of additional unsuspecting Americans are living potentially dangerous, stressful lives.

America's Mental Health Survey 2001[85] indicated that a staggering 88 million Americans were then experiencing symptoms related to mental health disorders, such as clinical depression and generalized stress disorders. The survey also noted that this was the case even though few people had ever been diagnosed with either disorder. Only those few who had been diagnosed showed up in other statistics. With this in mind, it is apparent that many Americans—and surely many other people of the world as well—are overburdened with preventable and treatable mental disorders such as depression, stress, and stress-related disorders, and need help now.

Depression, stress, and brain chemistry. Various physiological mechanisms occurring in the human organism may explain what causes depression and stress. After all, most cases of these disorders stem, at least in part, from insufficient levels of neurotransmitters in the brain.

One such neurotransmitter is serotonin, which research has found to be key to regulating our moods.[86,87] Serotonin was first discovered and isolated in the gastrointestinal tract in 1933. During 1947, it was discovered in blood platelets, and soon thereafter, it was found in the brain. (Scientists now realize that about 1 percent to 2 percent of serotonin exists there.) A few years later, in the 1950s, researchers began to recognize serotonin's effect on mood regulation. They found that people with sufficient serotonin levels were happier and more productive.[87,88,89] And since that time, serotonin has been referred to in some 78,000 studies published in scientific journals, making it one of the most investigated chemicals in the human system.[90]

The serotonin found in the brain, along with the 50 other neurotransmitters that have been identified so far, is produced by trillions of neurons (nerve cells). Each neuron is separated from the others by tiny gaps, called synapses. Serotonin and the other neurotransmitters allow the neurons to communicate by temporarily crossing synapses. And, in fact, scientists estimate that there are about one quadrillion synapses in the brain, and that each of the trillions of neurons in the brain can have as many as 10,000 synapses.[91,92,93]

Communication occurs when neurons produce and release neurotransmitters, which cross synapses and deliver chemical signals to other neurons. The synaptic gap between the neurons is only about one-millionth of an inch across, and neurotransmitters bridge the communication gap for only a few one-thousands of a second before decomposing or being absorbed into nerve endings. Still, every thought and positive or negative emotion we have is the result of millions of these chemical signals. Thus, an insufficient volume of a neurotransmitter such as serotonin results in inadequate chemical signaling, which manifests itself as an unhealthy state of mind.[87,89,91-95]

A number of stimuli cause serotonin levels to drop. First, serotonin can be depleted by traumatic life events and often it is following one, or a series of, traumatic event(s) that many people first experience depression or stress disorders. In addition, tobacco smoke, alcohol, herbicides, pesticides, nitrites, iodine, and physical stress can adversely affect neurotransmitter levels.[55,89] Of course, some people are also born with low levels of serotonin, and therefore, they are predisposed to become emotionally depressed or stressed more easily than others.[32,86] And, as previously described, serotonin levels have also been shown to decline with age,[96] which may explain why the first episode of depression typically occurs between the ages of 25 and 44, and why the incidence of depression increases with age.[35]

Antidepressant drugs and other substances generally extend the amount of time that serotonin and/or other neurotransmitters remain in the synapses, interacting with neurons.[87,97] Most antidepressants do so by blocking the neurotransmitters' decomposition or by preventing neurotransmitters from exiting into nerve endings. Both actions increase the amount of neurotransmitters in the brain, and by doing so, they should alleviate the symptoms of depression and stress disorders.[87,98,99]

However, successful treatment with prescription antidepressants often doesn't occur easily. In fact, *America's Mental Health Survey 2001* indicated that 54 percent of Americans who had taken antidepressant medication had also asked their doctors to change their medication at some point. And of the 54 percent who asked to be switched, 50 percent of patients said it was because of negative side effects, 28 percent said their antidepressant medication was not effective, and 18 percent said their antidepressant made them feel worse.[85]

Rhodiola rosea, depression, and stress. The good news is that in many cases *Rhodiola rosea* may offer a natural alternative to common medications for the prevention and treatment of depression and stress-related disorders. Unlike prescription drugs, it rarely brings adverse side effects, but like prescription antidepressant drugs, *Rhodiola rosea* protects serotonin and other neurotransmitters from depletion. It also enhances the availability of chemicals needed to produce serotonin. This results in increased serotonin levels in the brain and the alleviation of depression and stress.[55] As Zakir Ramazanov, Ph.D., along with Richard P. Brown, M.D., Associate Clinical Professor of Psychiatry at Columbia University College of Physicians and Surgeons, and Patricia L. Gerbarg, M.D., Assistant Clinical Professor in Psychiatry at New York Medical Center, stated in the scientific monograph *Rhodiola rosea: A Phytomedicinal Overview:* [In studies] "Overall, in small and medium doses, *Rhodiola rosea* stimulated norephinephrine, dopamine, serotonin, and nicotinic cholinergic effects in the central nervous system. It also enhanced the effects of these neurotransmitters on the brain by increasing the permeability of the blood brain barrier to precursors of dopamine and serotonin."[11]

It is this production and support of healthy brain chemistry that makes *Rhodiola rosea* so effective at fighting depression and stress-related disorders. In their book, Drs. Ramazanov and del Mar Bernal Suarez noted the following: "*Rhodiola rosea*'s proven effectiveness at treating depression and stress-related disorders has led Russian doctors to use it alone and sometimes in combination with antidepressants. By either method of application, the general intellectual and physical productivity levels of patients increased, while their lengths of stay in hospitals decreased. Furthermore, side effects normally associated with tricyclic antidepressants were lessened when the antidepressants were used in combination with *Rhodiola rosea*."[30,100] Earlier, Dr. Ramazanov and clinical nutritionist Carl Germano wrote in *Arctic Root [Rhodiola Rosea]: The Powerful New Ginseng Alternative* that *Rhodiola rosea* has proven itself to be a "safe and effective adjunct to conventional antidepressant therapy."[101] It has also been found to be an effective antistress and antidepression nutritional substance for everyday use.[1,2,101]

The positive effects of *Rhodiola rosea* may not be as pronounced as those sometimes produced by antidepressant and anti-anxiety drugs, however the results are significant as will be revealed in the following sections.

MENTAL DISORDERS

In one of many Soviet studies, a team of scientists led by Professor E. D. Krasik, M.D., of the Siberian State Medical University in Tomsk, Russia, observed the effect of *Rhodiola rosea* extract on 128 depressed individuals between the ages of 17 and 55.[102] Each patient was given the equivalent of about 100 milligrams of *Rhodiola rosea* extract twice a day for between one and four months. In the end, 64 percent of the patients showed substantial decreases in the clinical manifestations of their depression, and many patients' manifestations of depression completely disappeared. In these patients, *Rhodiola rosea* was shown to alleviate fatigue, irritability, distractibility, headache, weakness, and other vegetative symptoms.[30] And these subjective improvements were later confirmed by psychological testing and increased work productivity.[29,30,102]

While doing doctoral research in Moscow, Soviet scientist M. N. Mikhaylova studied the influence of *Rhodiola rosea* extract on 28 patients who suffered from asthenic syndromes. Each patient was given the equivalent of about 150 milligrams of *Rhodiola rosea* extract three times per day for between one and four months. In all 28 patients, general weakness, abnormal exhaustion in the mornings, daytime sleepiness, and abnormal fatigability decreased or disappeared. However, it should be noted that on the third day of treatment, one patient did experience anxiety and sleep disturbances. These effects were eliminated by reducing that patient's dose of *Rhodiola rosea* extract to about 60 milligrams twice per day.[29]

Dr. Mikhaylova also studied the effect of a higher dose of *Rhodiola rosea* extract in patients who suffered from asthenic syndromes. In this part of the study, 30 patients were administered the equivalent of about 250 milligrams of *Rhodiola rosea* extract three times per day for one to four months. Although the positive effects of *Rhodiola rosea* extract appeared more rapidly in these patients, a number of the patients receiving the higher doses experienced an increase in blood pressure, accompanied by squeezing pains in the chest during the second to third week of the study. Based on this observation, Dr. Mikhaylova recommended that treatment with large doses of *Rhodiola rosea* extract should be reduced as the symptoms of asthenic syndromes decline. Nonetheless, of all 58 patients, both those who received 150 milligrams doses or 250 milligrams doses of *Rhodiola rosea* extract, the majority exhibited improvements in their moods as their symptoms of asthenic syndromes declined. Furthermore, the patients became more sociable and active, their motivational levels increased, concentration and memory improved, and loud sounds and bright light did not cause stimulation, headache, or the sense of heaviness in the head that had occurred prior to treatment with *Rhodiola rosea* extract. Additionally, sleep improved for the majority of the 39 patients in the study who had difficulty falling asleep or achieving uninterrupted sleep prior to treatment with *Rhodiola rosea* extract.[29]

The renown pharmacologist Albert S. Saratikov, M.D., and biologist Efim A. Krasnov, D.Sc., professors at the Siberian State Medical University in Tomsk, Russia, report that in addition to lessening or eliminating symptoms of depression, clinical study has demonstrated that *Rhodiola rosea* extract lessens or eliminates symptoms of hypochondria that frequently accompany asthenic syndromes. *Rhodiola rosea* extract also has been proven to be effective in the treatment of several other neuroses as well, examples of which follow.[29]

In a Soviet study, 412 patients who suffered from asthenic syndromes and neuroses, as well as 53 healthy individuals were examined. In this study, doctors administered 50 milligrams of *Rhodiola rosea* three times per day for between ten days and four months. The result? The subjects' sluggishness decreased, their appetites improved, they expanded their

spheres of interests, their intellectual and physical work productivity increased, and they appeared to feel more cheerful
and vivacious.[29,30,102,102]

In yet another study, Professor Albert S. Saratikov, M.D.,
and colleagues reported how other patients who were suffering from neuroses showed marked improvements after being
treated with *Rhodiola rosea* extract. Prior to treatment, the 65
patients in the study complained of insomnia, increased irritability, and various physical disturbances. All were diagnosed
with various neuroses. These patients were prescribed 100
milligrams of *Rhodiola rosea* extract three times a day for 10
days. After 10 days, the patients appeared to be more alert,
their reflexes and concentration improved, and they were
better able to distinguish between positive and negative stimuli. In addition, the patients' verbal responses came more
quickly, and their attention spans and memories improved.
And finally, the patients became less verbose and gave far
more meaningful responses to questions.[29,30,104,105]

In a study conducted between 1981 and 1986, Drs. V. Y.
Semko and V. N. Sudakov of the Scientific Research Institute
of Psychiatry of the Soviet Academy of Medical Sciences in
Tomsk also showed that *Rhodiola rosea* was beneficial in
treating mental disturbances. They looked specifically at disturbances resulting from trauma and vascular lesions of the
brain. In the end, these researchers found that *Rhodiola rosea*
produced the best results in patients whose treatment began
as they were just beginning to develop nervous and mental
disturbances.[30,106]

Professors Albert S. Saratikov, M.D., and Efim A. Krasnov,
D.Sc., recommend that *Rhodiola rosea* extract also should be
used in treatment of asthenia/depression associated with certain forms of schizophrenia. Their research shows that following administration of *Rhodiola rosea* extract, patients suf-

fering from asthenia and periodic and paranoid forms of schizophrenia experienced less sluggishness, expanded their spheres of interests, increased their intellectual and physical work productivity, and noticed the apprearance of feelings of cheerfulness and vivacity.[29]

Professor Albert S. Saratikov, M.D., reported that *Rhodiola rosea* extract can also relieve some mental disturbances caused by adverse health conditions of the body. What are these conditions? Well, for example, feelings of depression and fatigue can also be caused by low blood pressure, or malfunctioning adrenal or thyroid glands.[107-111] And nervousness and shakiness that may mimick anxiety disorders, can actually be caused by malfunctioning adrenal or thyroid glands as well.[108,110] *Rhodiola rosea*'s effectiveness in ameliorating the nonpsychiatric causes of these symptoms has been demonstrated in either clinical or laboratory research. In a clinical study performed at the Siberian State Medical University in Tomsk, Russia, Dr. A. P. Faeeva treated 177 patients suffering from hypotension (low blood pressure) with *Rhodiola rosea* extract. The result? Ninety-two percent of the patients experienced "stable, full, or partial normalization" of blood pressure levels. In further detailing the results of the study, Professor Albert S. Saratikov stated that the hypotensive patients who responded to *Rhodiola rosea* extract therapy experienced "an improvement in well-being, disappearance of headaches, normalization of sleep, and [their] recovery of work capacity ensued concurrently."[29]

Professors Albert S. Saratikov, M.D., and Efim A. Krasnov, D.Sc., have also performed research on *Rhodiola rosea* extract's effectiveness in preventing and treating dysfunctions of the endocrine system—dysfunctions that could produce feelings of depression and fatigue as well as nervousness and shakiness normally indicative of anxiety disorders. In translating this research, Professor Zakir Ramazanov, Ph.D., of Spain's University of Las Palmas stated that Drs. Saratikov and Krasnovs' studies demonstrate that *Rhodiola rosea* extract "enhances thyroid function without causing hyperthyroidism [a condition marked by enlargement of the thyroid gland, rapid heart rate, high blood pressure, etc.], enhances thymus gland function and protects and delays involution [shriveling of the thymus gland] that occurs with aging. [*Rhodiola rosea* extract also] improves adrenal gland reserves, without causing hypertrophy [overgrowth of the organ]."[30]

Protecting and improving the performance of the adrenal, thymus and thyroid glands—as *Rhodiola rosea* extract has been shown to do—should help prevent psychiatric-like symptoms that could otherwise be produced by dysfunction of these vital endocrine organs.

Based on these studies, it is clear that *Rhodiola rosea* has the power to significantly improve people's mental health and well-being. But *Rhodiola rosea* can also improve people's mental/intellectual performance, as we'll explore next.

MENTAL PERFORMANCE

Thanks to its power as both a psychostimulant and an adaptogen, *Rhodiola rosea* extract has been shown to improve people's mental performance in a variety of ways. It also has helped people who prematurely weaken while performing work—especially intellectual work—and it has helped fight so-called "afternoon tiredness." *Rhodiola rosea*'s positive effects on mental performance are documented in numerous scientific studies.

For example, in a study conducted for the Russian Ministry of Health in Moscow, a team of scientists headed by Dr. V. A. Shevtsov measured the effect of a single dose of *Rhodiola rosea* extract on the mental performance of 161 Russian cadets.[112] The cadets were all males between the ages of 19 and 21, and all were in good mental and physical shape. And, all had been well-trained to be able to cope with physical and mental strain and stress. At the outset of the study, each cadet was evaluated on how quickly he could complete a specific task, the quantity and quality of his task performance, his short-term memory capacity, and his ability to maintain focus or switch focus when necessary. Then, each cadet completed a questionnaire and was randomly chosen as a member of one of four groups. Group 1 received 370 milligrams of *Rhodiola rosea* extract. Group 2 received 555 milligrams of the extract. Group 3 received a placebo, and Group 4 was the control group. The capsules were taken at 4 a.m. while the cadets were in the middle of a 24-hour schedule of routine military service, including night duty. Then, one hour after the capsules were consumed, each cadet was retested and reexamined, and each completed another questionnaire.

Test results reveal that the placebo and control groups performed almost identically. And while there was virtually no improvement in the average mental performance of the placebo and control groups after treatment, there was a dramatic and significant improvement in the average mental performance of cadets who consumed *Rhodiola rosea* extract. These cadet groups experienced less fatigue, and their average capacity for mental work was 13.75 percent greater than that of the placebo group. Furthermore, an analysis of the cadets' questionnaires revealed that while only 11.25 percent of the cadets in the placebo and control groups felt better two hours after treatment, 49 percent of the cadets who consumed *Rhodiola rosea* extract felt better after treatment.[112]

In another study, students between the ages of twenty and twenty-eight performed a proofreading test based on the

Anfimov table—a standard table that allows one to compare the quality and quantity of work performed. The students were then given either a *Rhodiola rosea* solution or a similar-looking placebo.[30,113] One hour after taking the placebo, that group's members made 13 percent more errors in their work. By the fourth hour, placebo group errors had increased 37 percent. By the sixth hour, 88 percent, and by the eighth hour, 180 percent. In contrast, after taking *Rhodiola rosea*, the other group's errors decreased by 56 percent, and these group members were able to maintain this level of work quality for four hours. After four hours, the group's error percentage began to increase, but to a lesser extent than the placebo group.[30,113]

Rhodiola rosea extract's effects on mental performance were again studied on twenty-seven healthy student physicians and scientists, who ranged in age from nineteen to forty-six. Once or twice per day, beginning several days before the students completed some intense intellectual work, researchers gave the group between 100 milligrams and 150 milligrams of *Rhodiola rosea* extract. The effect? The students completed more work than normal and better work, and their work activity was not curtailed by fatigue.[30,103]

In other research, Drs. V. Darbinyan and A. Kteyan of the Armenian State Medical University along with other scientists studied the effects of *Rhodiola rosea* extract on physicians who had been assigned to prolonged night duty. Thirty-three of the physicians were female, twenty-three were male, all were in good health, and all ranged in age from twenty-four to thirty-five. Each of the fifty-six physicians in the study took five different tests on complex perceptive and cognitive cerebral functions, such as associative thinking, short-term memory, calculation and concentration abilities, and speed of audiovisual perception. The tests were taken both before and after night duty during three two-week periods and measured each physician's mental performance and fatigue. At the end of this double-blind trial, the twenty-six physicians who received 170 milligrams of *Rhodiola rosea* extract per day showed a statistically significant improvement in mental performance when compared to the thirty physicians who received identical-looking placebo capsules. However, *Rhodiola rosea*'s positive effects ended by the sixth week, probably because of the low dosage used and/or the length of the strenuous night duty.[4]

In another double-blind, placebo-controlled study, this one conducted for the Russian Ministry of Public Health, Drs. A. A. Spasov, V. B. Mandrikov and I. A. Mironova tested the effects of *Rhodiola rosea* extract on sixty high school students. The students who received *Rhodiola rosea* extract exhibited improvements in physical work capacity, coordination, and general well being, and they had less mental fatigue and situational anxiety.[114]

And finally, in yet another double-blind, placebo-controlled study, a group of Indian students studying medicine at the Volgograd State Medical Academy were given 100 milligrams of *Rhodiola rosea* extract per day during their final exam period. The students who received *Rhodiola rosea* extract exhibited significant improvements in well-being, physical fitness, coordination, and even final exam grades, and they had less mental fatigue compared to the placebo group.[115]

Clearly, then, given the abundance of scientific data, *Rhodiola rosea* extract has proven itself as a powerful tool against mental fatigue. It has been shown to improve mental performance in nearly everyone who uses it, thanks to its stimulative and adaptogenic properties.

Beyond mental performance, though, the plant also makes

a difference in physical performance and energy levels. Next, we'll discuss these benefits in more detail.

PHYSICAL PERFORMANCE

Each person's physical performance depends on energy. So to begin our discussion of *Rhodiola rosea*'s energy-enhancing properties, let's examine how the body produces energy.

Normally, our cells' mitochondria use glucose to produce energy. However, although glucose is the easiest and fastest energy source for the body, it is a relatively poor energy source, as are the carbohydrates that convert to glucose. In actuality, the richest energy source is fatty acids, since fatty acids play a greater role in supporting the body's energy demands long term than glucose.[30,116]

Now, Russian scientists have shown that *Rhodiola rosea* can increase the amount of fatty acids in the blood. This may partly explain how the plant enhances physical performance, increases endurance, and quickens recovery from fatigue.[30]

In addition to increasing fatty acid levels, *Rhodiola rosea* also helps the body complete the tasks fatty acids are designed to do. Normally, when they are metabolized in cellular mitochondria, fatty acids are converted into energy that is used to produce ATP and creatine phosphate. Now, researchers at Tomsk State Medicinal Sciences University have shown that *Rhodiola rosea* stimulates ATP and creatine phosphate production in muscle tissue, which thereby increases energy levels. In these researchers' studies, improvements in eyesight and motor coordination followed.[25,30,117]

Additionally, scientists at the Russian Institute for Highest Sports Achievements have compared *Rhodiola rosea* extract with common anabolic steroids. They found *Rhodiola rosea*'s effects on physical performance to be comparable to steroid compounds, yet *Rhodiola rosea* had none of the negative effects on adrenal cortex function that steroids produce. Also, anabolic steroids' other effects, including the enhancement of male sexual characteristics, were not seen in patients who took *Rhodiola rosea* extract.[30,118]

Truly, there is an abundance of scientific research on *Rhodiola rosea* extract's ability to enhance physical performance, but I'll give just one more example of this. In another study conducted by Tomsk State University scientists, 112 Soviet athletes were given either *Rhodiola rosea* or a placebo prior to competing in track and field, swimming, speed skating, or skiing. As a result, 89 percent of the athletes who received *Rhodiola rosea* extract showed improved physical performances, more rapid passing of fatigue, and less apathy after physical exertion than the placebo group, and 69 percent adapted to climatic and social conditions faster than the placebo group. Additionally, by the end of the study, the athletes who had taken *Rhodiola rosea* extract showed improvements in general health. Their pulse rates were better, their arterial pressure was lower, their lungs showed increased vital capacity, their back muscles were stronger, their hands were better able to endure static tension, they were more coordinated in their movements, their recovery periods were shorter, and the time it took for their heart rates and arterial pressure to normalize had gone down. Side effects such as palpitations, sleep disturbances, and loss of appetite, were not observed.[30,119]

Last, another way *Rhodiola rosea* extract enhances physical performance and protects athletes is by inhibiting free radical production during exercise. Normally, strenuous physical exercise increases the production of free radicals, which can result in cell damage, muscle injury, and cholesterol oxidation.[120-124] But thanks to its antioxidant activity, *Rhodiola rosea* extract has been shown to inhibit the production of damaging free radicals and repair damage caused by free radicals.[125] Clearly, *Rhodiola rosea* extract is a boon to physical fitness.

WEIGHT MANAGEMENT

As you might expect, while enhancing physical perform-ance, *Rhodiola rosea* can also help with weight management. To explain this role, though, we must return to the discussion of dietary fat that we began in Chapter 3.

To reiterate, fat is an essential part of good health because it plays a crucial role in helping our brains operate normally, in building cell membranes, and in producing energy.[126] But at the same time, fat can cause problems when too much is consumed. High fat intake causes people to be overweight and obese and is responsible for increasing the onset poten-tial and severity of cardiovascular diseases, diabetes, gallblad-der disease, osteoarthritis, certain cancers, and other disor-ders. And people who are obese have a 50 percent to 100 percent higher risk of death from all causes than normal-weight individuals.[127]

In order to be absorbed into the body and stored or finally used, dietary fat must first be broken down into free fatty acids. This is done with the help of a key enzyme: pancreatic lipase. The resulting free fatty acids then cross intestinal membranes and are absorbed, and after absorption, they are distributed throughout the body with blood flow. Some of the fatty acids then break down in the mitochondria to pro-duce vital energy, but the remaining, unutilized fatty acids accumulate in adipose (fat) tissue.[128-131]

Eliminating pancreatic lipase or blocking its activity would mean that dietary fat would not be absorbed into the body. Instead, it would simply pass through the body. Therefore,

Table 15. Percent of fatty acid released into
blood serum during resting conditions

Time	0	60 Minutes
Placebo Group	100%	102±1.3%
Rhodiola Rosea Group	100%	109±2.1%

Source: Zakir Ramazanov, Ph.D., 2001.[30]

partially blocking pancreatic lipase activity, as *Rhododendron caucasicum* has been shown to do, reduces the amount of fat that is absorbed which results in weight loss.[30,132]

But what about the fat that has already been stored in adipose tissue? Well, as noted previously, *Rhododendron caucasicum* both inhibits pancreatic lipase and activates a lipase enzyme called hormone sensitive lipase to break up fat in adipose tissue. However, in this latter function, *Rhodiola rosea* is even more effective.[1]

Rhodiola rosea is extremely successful at activating hormone sensitive lipase, which breaks down and liberates fat

Table 16. Percent of fatty acid released into blood serum
following 1 hour of bicycle exercise

Time	0	60 Minutes
Placebo Group	100%	119±1.2%
Rhodiola Rosea Group	100%	172±2.7%

Source: Zakir Ramazanov, Ph.D., 2001.[30]

Table 17. Percent of fatty acid released into blood serum
following 30 minutes of normal walking

Time	0	30 Minutes
Placebo Group	100%	104±1.1%
Rhodiola Rosea Group	100%	122±1.2%

Source: Zakir Ramazanov, Ph.D., 2001.[30]

from adipose tissue. The released fatty acids then circulate in the blood and eventually enter cells' mitochondria to produce energy. To lose weight, then, one must burn off the fatty acids immediately after they are released. This can be done through simple exercise.[30] Interestingly, exercise also activates hormone sensitive lipase, releasing more fat from adipose tissue. So exercising after consuming *Rhodiola rosea* produces a volume of fat release far greater than can be achieved by either *Rhodiola rosea* or exercise alone.[1]

Research on Rhodiola rosea and weight management. More than thirty years of Soviet scientific research has proven *Rhodiola rosea* extract's effectiveness in weight management. Specifically, these studies have demonstrated the extract's ability to activate hormone sensitive lipase and release fatty acids from adipose tissue.

In one Soviet clinical study on fatty acid release, researchers administered either a placebo or *Rhodiola rosea* extract to 121 healthy volunteers between the ages of 23 and 65.[30]After the volunteers had rested one hour, the researchers took blood samples from each of them and analyzed the blood. The result was that, even when patients were resting,

Rhodiola rosea extract increased the amount of fatty acids released into their bloodstreams.

Then, during a second phase of the same study, new blood samples from the same 121 healthy volunteers were analyzed after the volunteers completed one hour of bicycle exercise.[30] And while exercise alone increased the amount of fatty acids released into the volunteers' bloodstreams, the combination of *Rhodiola rosea* extract and exercise tremendously increased this amount.

In another clinical study on fatty acid release, patients were divided into two groups. The first group of 137 people received placebo capsules, while the second group of 133 people received 200 milligrams of *Rhodiola rosea* extract. After the patients completed 30 minutes of moderate walking, each gave a blood sample, which was then analyzed. This time the result, again, was that while exercise alone increased the amount of fatty acids released into the bloodstream, the combination of *Rhodiola rosea* extract and exercise increased the amount even more.[30,133,134]

Rhodiola rosea extract's effect on weight reduction and fat metabolism was also examined at Georgian State Hospital in Tblisi.[30] In this study, 273 obese patients were divided into two groups. One group of 70 men and 60 women was given 300 milligrams of *Rhodiola rosea* extract before each meal, three times a day. The control group of 143 patients was given identical-looking placebos at identical times. All the test subjects were then instructed to select foods from a regular menu, but they were advised to limit their caloric intake. They were also restricted from eating sweets or fast food. And 60 minutes after completing their meals, the patients were required to walk for 30 to 40 minutes. The result was that in the group taking *Rhodiola rosea* extract, the average weight of 175 pounds at the beginning of the test dropped to 154.5

pounds by the end of the 90-day test period. All told, 92 percent of these patients lost weight. In addition, their average
body fat ratio decreased to 25.14 percent from the 31.07 percent it had been at the start of the test. The patients' general
health improved, as did their moods and sleep patterns.

In commenting on this study, Dr. Zakir Ramazanov, noted,
"It is interesting that the placebo group also experienced
weight reduction. Their weight dropped from an average of
173 pounds to 165 pounds. The weight reduction exhibited
by the placebo group shows what some dietary common
sense and simple exercise can do for people."[30,133]

***Rhodiola rosea* and *Rhododendron caucasicum* together.** Based
on the aforementioned research, it is obvious that *Rhodiola
rosea* is particularly effective at helping with weight loss.
However, research also shows that taking it along with
Rhododendron caucasicum is even more effective.

One study in particular showed that certain women who
simultaneously took *Rhodiola rosea* extract and *Rhododendron
caucasicum* extract experienced exceptional weight loss.
Professor Musa T. Abidoff, M.D., of the Moscow Center for
Modern Medicine, conducted the study on 45 women
between the ages of 21 and 42. On average, the women were
35.2 years old and weighed 164.5 pounds. Each had delivered
a child and finished lactation at least four months before the
tests began. For eight weeks, each woman was given 200 milligrams of *Rhodiola rosea* extract and 100 milligrams of
Rhododendron caucasicum extract three times a day. In the
end, the researchers noted that for the first six weeks, average
weight reduction was gradual (5 percent to 6 percent), but by
the last two weeks, average weight loss increased to 14 percent. During the same eight-week period, the patients' body
fat ratios dropped. Fat around their waists decreased by an

average 11.5 percent, while bust sizes decreased by 5 percent on average.[134]

These results, along with numerous others cited in this book, demonstrate these plants' power in ensuring good health. But let's return to the specific benefits that can come from taking *Rhodiola rosea* alone, because in addition to helping with mental and physical performance and weight reduction, this plant protects against heart damage, particularly from arrhythmias.

ARRHYTHMIA

First, some background. As noted previously, one of the ills that make stress particularly dangerous is its ability to damage the heart. Among other methods of causing such damage, stress stimulates the release of chemicals called catecholamines—the most famous of which is adrenaline—into the bloodstream. Catecholamines are dangerous because they can cause blood vessels to constrict, increase blood pressure and play a role in the development of hypertension, make blood more prone to clotting (thereby increasing the risk of an arterial blockage and heart attack or stroke), and increase the pulse and the force of heart contractions. And during stressful events, catecholamines cause the heart to contract with such severe intensity that it creates microscopic tears in muscle fibers of the heart. These wounds are called contraction band lesions.

Contraction band lesions are made up of dead cells, and when they are present, they cause a disruption in the electrical impulses that normally flow through healthy heart muscle and cause the heart to contract (beat). Because it is then unable to receive the correct electrical impulses, the heart eventually begins beating out of sequence—a phenomenon known as an arrhythmia. Major arrhythmias can prevent the heart and other areas of the body from receiving enough oxygen, which can cause cardiac arrest.[81,83,135-139]

Many people believe sudden cardiac deaths (unexpected fatal heart attacks) are caused by arterial blood clots, but the fact is, about 86 percent of these deaths result from "toxic doses of catecholamines (adrenaline and noradrenaline) prescribed by the angry brain," according to researcher and clinician Naras Bhat, M.D.[136] In fact, a single stressful event can produce catecholamine-induced heart contractions severe enough to create and rupture a contraction band lesion and instantly stop the heart. Catecholamine overloads are not always immediately heart-stopping, however. Sometimes it takes years of chronic and/or repeated stress-induced catecholamine overloads to damage the heart muscle enough to disrupt its electrical impulses. Eventually, though, the ensuing arrhythmias, reductions in the heart's pumping power, and oxygen deprivation to the heart will stop the heart from beating. Therefore, whether the effects of uncontrolled stress manifest themselves immediately or after several years, the end result is death.[136]

Fortunately, research has demonstrated that *Rhodiola rosea* extract prevents stress-induced damage to the heart.[24,27,140] Teams of scientists at the Russian Academy of Medical Sciences in Tomsk, Russia, have shown that *Rhodiola rosea* extract prevents stress-induced catecholamine release in heart muscle and have demonstrated that the extract can prevent high levels of the chemical cyclic-AMP from accumulating in the heart.[25,28] Limiting cyclic-AMP is important because cyclic-AMP can increases the heart's contraction rate during stressful events.[141,142] In other research, *Rhodiola rosea* extract has also been shown to prevent arrhythmias induced by adrenaline or calcium chloride in animals.[27,28]

HEARING

In addition to protecting the heart, *Rhodiola rosea* can also protect our hearing, as scientific studies have shown. For example, Vladimir F. Oleynichenko, M.D., an assistant professor at the All-Russian Research Institute of Medicine and Medical-Technical Information in Tomsk, Russia, investigated *Rhodiola rosea* extract's effect on the auditory organs of twenty-two healthy individuals. Three of the subjects were pilots at a Soviet airport. The other nineteen worked in an electromechanical production plant, where the noise intensity was between 100 and 180 decibels.[143,144]

Prior to treatment, Dr. Oleynichenko evaluated these subjects' perception of whispered and conversational speech and conducted tuning fork and tonal audiometer tests. He measured air and bone conduction through earphones (air) and through a vibrator that had been placed on the mastoid bone behind the

Table 18. Sound Volume and Effects on Hearing

Sound	Volume in Decibels	Comparable Loudness
Absolute silence	0	
A light whisper	10	Base
A busy street	70	10 million times louder
Probable Permanent Hearing Loss With Repeated Exposure		
A subway	90 (to 100)	1 billion times louder
Extreme Danger		
A jet airport	120	1 trillion times louder
A close-up jet engine	150	1 quadrillion times louder

Source: Texas Workers' Compensation Commission, 1998,2003.[145]

ear (bone). With this test, a lower conduction reading correlated to a decrease in hearing ability, and after giving it, Dr. Oleynichenko identified a decrease in air and bone conduction for speech tones in all twenty-two subjects. In other words, all twenty-two subjects had a hard time hearing speech tones.

Following the examination, each patient was given 100 milligrams of *Rhodiola rosea* extract twice a day for two to three weeks. And by the end of the second week, air and bone conduction for speech tones increased in all twenty-two individuals—10 to 20 decibels in twenty subjects, and 30 to 40 decibels in two subjects. In other words, all of the subjects began to hear speech better—some a great deal better. For high tones, air conduction increased by 10 decibels in nine subjects and by 30 to 40 decibels in three subjects, but it remained unchanged in 10 individuals. And bone conduction for all tones increased 10 to 30 decibels in nine subjects and remained unchanged in thirteen. So not only did the *Rhodiola rosea* extract help the subjects hear speech tones better, but it also helped some of them hear high-pitched sounds and everything else better, too.[143,144]

But again, the plant's effectiveness isn't limited to any particular organ, whether the ears or the heart. Its efficacies extend throughout the body. For instance, *Rhodiola rosea* can also protect against cancer, which we'll discuss next.

CANCER

As described previously, cells routinely reproduce themselves by dividing—a process called mitosis—but a problem can occur when the mechanisms that regulate cells' rate of mitosis are damaged. Suddenly, the cell is free to reproduce itself without restraint, and when it does so exponentially, the result is cancer.

Also, when a single cell first begins to replicate at an abnormal rate, it is usually the result of DNA damage in that cell. Most often, this damage is caused by free radicals, especially carcinogenic chemicals and physical agents, such as ultraviolet light and radiation.[146–154]

Fortunately, *Rhodiola rosea* is rich in free radical neutralizers, which protect and repair cells and their DNA, thus inhibiting the onset and progression of cancer.[19,125] In addition, the plant is a potent detoxifier and regenerator of the liver.[22,155] And since liver damage (and damage to immune system cells) often occurs in people who are suffering from cancer or who are being treated with anticancer drugs, *Rhodiola rosea* can be said to help fight cancer's effects in several ways.

But let's examine these effects in more detail. First, in animal studies, *Rhodiola rosea* has been shown to enhance cancer drugs while simultaneously reducing some of their side effects.[22,155] For example, in one study, tumor cells were transplanted into two groups of mice.[11,22,30] As intended, one group of mice developed Ehrlich adenocarcinoma, a cancer of the glandular tissues, and the other group of mice developed Lewis lung cancer. The mice then were treated with the cancer drug cyclophosphamide, which suppressed tumor growth by as much as 39 percent and also limited metastases (spreading) of cancer cells to 18 percent. But the cyclophosphamide also produced a side effect: it reduced the mice's white blood cell count to 40 percent of normal and their bone marrow cell count to 20 percent of normal.

In contrast, in mice that were given both *Rhodiola rosea* extract and the cancer drug, cyclophosphamide, the effect was notable. *Rhodiola rosea* extract increased cyclophosphamide's suppression of metastases 36 percent, increased the number of white blood cells 30 percent, and increased the number of bone marrow cells as much as 18 percent. In addition, in mice that were treated with *Rhodiola rosea* extract alone, the extract suppressed tumor growth by between 19 percent and 27 percent, and it suppressed metastases of Lewis lung cancer by 16 percent. Furthermore, it caused no reduction in the number of white blood cells or bone marrow cells.[11,22,30]

Additional studies have also demonstrated *Rhodiola rosea*'s effectiveness against cancer. In another study, this one on mice suffering from cancerous tumors, *Rhodiola rosea* extract increased the effectiveness of the cancer drug adriamycin and dramatically reduced the liver-damaging side effects of the drug.[21] Also, in an experiment on rats suffering from Pliss lymphosarcoma, a cancer that originates in the lymphatic system, *Rhodiola rosea* extract, given alone, inhibited tumor growth by 39 percent and inhibited metastases by 50 percent.[22] And finally, in a small initial human study, scientists observed *Rhodiola rosea* extract's effect on patients suffering from superficial bladder cancer. The extract improved the integrity of tissue in the urinary tract, boosted immunity, and reduced the frequency of relapses.[156]

AMENORRHEA

Rhodiola rosea can also help with amenorrhea, the absence of menstrual periods. This condition can result from the late onset of puberty, or it can be caused by obesity, extreme weight loss, excessive exercise, stress, medications, contraceptives, and disorders of the uterus, ovaries, pituitary gland, and/or hypothalamus.[157]

In a Soviet study, Dr. N. D. Gerasimova of the Siberian State Medical University in Tomsk, Russia, tested *Rhodiola rosea* extract's effectiveness at treating amenorrhea. The doctor used the extract to treat 40 women between the ages of

19 and 35, all of whom had suffered from amenorrhea for five months to five-plus years. All of the patients received general clinical examinations and gynecological exams before and after treatment. Most were prescribed *Rhodiola rosea* extract totaling 100 milligrams to 200 milligrams per day, depending on the severity of their condition, for two weeks. The rest were given a daily injection of a 1 milliliter solution of *Rhodiola rosea* extract for 10 days. And for most patients, the particular treatment was repeated two or three times (in some cases as often as four times). The result was that, by the end of the study, 25 of the 40 women had normal menstrual cycles. Dr. Gerasimova also noted that the general physical condition of all the patients significantly improved, and 11 of the 25 patients with restored menstrual cycles became pregnant.[30,158]

ERECTILE DYSFUNCTION

Finally, in addition to helping women's reproductive organs and cycles, *Rhodiola rosea* can also enhance the function of male reproductive organs. For example, in clinical research, Dr. Alexander S. Kodkin, at Siberian State Medical University in Tomsk, Russia, found *Rhodiola rosea* extract to be a successful treatment for men who suffer from erectile dysfunction and/or premature ejaculation. In Dr. Kodkin's study, thirty-five patients who had been suffering from weak erection, premature ejaculation, or a combination thereof for between one and twenty years were observed. An overwhelming majority of these patients also complained of irritability, excitability, poor sleep, and sweatiness. So, *Rhodiola rosea* extract was prescribed: 100 milligrams to 200 milligrams a day for three months. The result? A substantial improvement in sexual function in 74 percent of the patients, including normalization of prostate fluid and an increase in male sex hormones.[30,159-162]

Choosing a Rhodiola Rosea Extract

Now that *Rhodiola rosea*'s benefits have been outlined, it is important to discuss what characteristics to look for in an extract of the plant. In particular, one should note that there are differences in phytochemical composition between various rhodiola species. In addition, use of the plant comes with a warning for anyone with bipolar disorder, as noted below.

PHYTOCHEMICAL COMPOSITION

There are at least twenty species of rhodiola, and pharmacological activity has warranted chemical analysis of sixteen of these species. Now, after years of experimentation, it is clear that only the species *Rhodiola rosea* produces the unique and powerful health-enhancing results described in this book.[30]

For example, Soviet pharmacologist Vladimir A. Kurkin, D.Sc., of Kujbyshev Medical Institute in Moscow and chemist Gertruda G. Zapesochnaya, D.Sc., of the Moscow Institute of Fine Chemical Technology have presented fourteen separate studies detailing how the chemical composition of *Rhodiola rosea* root is very different from other species of rhodiola.[30,163] They and other scientists, using the high performance liquid chromatography method of analysis, have demonstrated that only *Rhodiola rosea* root contains cinnamyl alcohol b-vicianoside rosavin, rosin, and rosarin—collectively called rosavins.[164,165] Rosavins have not been found in any other rhodiola species. And while salidroside, another key *Rhodiola rosea* component, was found in all other rhodiola species, only *Rhodiola rosea* produces both rosavins and salidroside.[1,30]

Based on the above analysis, along with other convincing evidence, the Russian Pharmacopoeia Committee adopted a new standard for *Rhodiola rosea* extract in 1989. The committee declared that *Rhodiola rosea* extract must contain both rosavins and salidroside in order to be identified as an extract of *Rhodiola rosea*.[166]

Rosavins and salidroside are key pharmacological components of *Rhodiola rosea*, and therefore, their volume is standardized in high-quality supplements. But further research also indicates that standardized extracts should contain all the other active constituents that are naturally found in *Rhodiola rosea* as well. In fact, including all of *Rhodiola rosea*'s constituents in a supplement has been shown to produce far superior physiological results than the extract's individual, purified components alone.[1,30] So be sure to find a supplement that contains all of *Rhodiola rosea*'s components.

In addition, *Rhodiola rosea* should never be diluted with other rhodiola species—all of which are pharmacologically inferior to *Rhodiola rosea*. In the late 1980s, some nutritional supplement makers attempted this in order to reduce costs and meet supply demands. The result was a dramatic decline in product quality and effectiveness. Fortunately, such attempts were abandoned long ago by ethical supplement producers.[1,30] However, even today, the unsuspecting public often purchases products labeled rhodiola under the mistaken assumption that rhodiola and *Rhodiola rosea* are the same substance. They are not, and this fact cannot be reiterated enough. Furthermore, all of the studies reported in this book—and, as of early 2003, approximately 51 percent of all animal rhodiola studies and 94 percent of all human rhodiola studies—were performed using the species *Rhodiola rosea.*[11] So, when choosing an extract, be sure to look for one made from *Rhodiola rosea*, not some other rhodiola species. This will help ensure that the extract is as effective as outlined here.

SAFETY AND CONTRAINDICATIONS

Finally, a quick note about safety. The species *Rhodiola rosea* has been found to be safe and nonaddicting for both animals and humans.[11] However, Richard P. Brown, M.D., Patricia L. Gerbarg, M.D., and Zakir Ramazanov, Ph.D., have stated in *Rhodiola Rosea: A Phytomedicinal Overview* that "*Rhodiola rosea* has an activating antidepressant effect, [and] it should not be used [by] individuals with bipolar disorder, who are vulnerable to becoming manic when given antidepressants or stimulants."[11] Consumers should certainly keep this warning in mind.

Ancient Wisdom, Modern Science

Overall, like the other plants described in this book, *Rhodiola rosea*'s safety and health-protecting benefits have been demonstrated during centuries of use in folk medicine. But even more important, the plant's safety and medicinal properties have been further demonstrated and confirmed in over 150 modern biochemical, toxicological, pharmacological, and clinical studies. These were performed at leading scientific research centers over the last forty-two years.

Today, *Rhodiola rosea*'s growing fame in the United States is mostly due to its ability to increase mental and physical performance, and to prevent and treat emotional stress and depression. Of course, as has been shown, the plant's additional efficacies are many, varied, and equally impressive. Among them, *Rhodiola rosea* has been shown to protect against free radical damage, enhance DNA repair, suppress tumor growth, help reduce metastasizing of certain cancers, lessen stress-induced damage to the heart, prevent arrhythmias, and regenerate the liver. All of these benefits slow the onset and progression of age-related diseases and aging itself, as long-living Georgians have shown.

As we conclude this chapter, one final thought seems pertinent. A total of four antiaging plants have been described in this book. Each of these plants provides its own unique and remarkable protection for the health of the entire body. However, in many cases, the plants' greatest protective and healing effects are specific to certain organs, systems, and illnesses. Therefore, to achieve maximum health and antiaging benefits, extracts of all four antiaging plants should become part of a daily nutritional regimen. Such has been the approach of others who have used these supplements and who can attest to their efficacy, as you will see in the book's Conclusion.

CHAPTER 7

Conclusion

This book is a testament to the sheer brilliance of the Georgian lifestyle and Georgian folk medicine, and the foresight of modern-day Georgian science. It is amazing that a single land could produce so much botanical wealth, and that its people could discover and implement so much medicinal good from that wealth. The intrinsic ingenuity and skill of Georgian practitioners, past and present, now provides unparalleled protection and treatment for the health of everyone living in this twenty-first century.

If we look only at the four Georgian folk medicines described in this book, we find nutritional abundance unrivaled anywhere else on earth. All four plants are powerful antioxidants and free radical neutralizers. All four limit DNA damage caused by carcinogens. All four are rich in nutrients that inhibit the onset and spread of cancers. All four slow the onset and progression of atherosclerosis. All four are rich in nutrients that protect cholesterol from free radical damage.

All four strengthen blood vessels in the brain and body. And all four protect against liver damage.

Now, add to those efficacies the fact that three of the four plants are rich in nutrients that protect brain cells from oxidation and death. Three of the four are active against certain pathogenic bacteria and viruses. Two of the four are powerful adaptogens. Two break up fat from adipose tissue. Two help normalize blood pressure and pulse. And individually, these plants reduce fat absorption, reduce sugar absorption and glucose synthesis, help prevent glaucoma, lower uric acid and prevent and treat gout, help prevent and treat depression, stress disorders, and neuroses, improve mental and physical performance, protect against stress-induced damage to the heart, and prevent heart arrhythmia.

Finally, consider that these important effects are supported by literally thousands of studies published in peer-reviewed scientific journals. All considered, it is easy to see the antiaging benefits awarded to people who consume these plants on a regular basis.

Reports from North Americans

The first Georgian medicinal plant extract to become available to North Americans was *Rhododendron caucasicum* extract. During late 1997, information about this plant and its benefits was sent to a few thousand Americans and Canadians, and shortly thereafter, *Rhododendron caucasicum* extract itself was made available for purchase on a limited basis. Because *Rhododendron caucasicum*'s effects can be quite subtle, few customers noticed any immediate benefits. Within three months, however, the benefits the extract produced became very apparent.

It all started with a call from a man named Ed Buckman. Ed was sixty-seven years old when he began taking *Rhododendron caucasicum* extract. He had given blood once every fifty-eight days for more than ten years, and for the previous three and a half years, the blood center had rewarded him for each of his donations with a free cholesterol test. Well, Ed had a dangerous total cholesterol level of at least 266 for most of his adult life. He was under the care of a physician, he ate a very low-cholesterol diet, and he exercised and did everything else possible to lower his cholesterol. However, despite all this, he'd only been able to lower his total cholesterol to 266.

I heard from Ed three months after he had started using *Rhododendron caucasicum* extract. To his surprise, his cholesterol had dropped sixty-nine points to 197 just by using the extract those few months. And what was even more remarkable was that he had three and a half years of cholesterol test results to prove his claims! Later, after six months of using *Rhododendron caucasicum* extract, Ed Buckman's total cholesterol dropped another fifty points to 147.

But Ed's was not the only success story to come my way. A colleague, Charles Olive, also reported great success with *Rhododendron caucasicum* extract. In order to manage a series of illnesses, physicians had performed complete physicals, including blood chemistry analyses, on Charles two to three times per year for more than eleven years. Throughout that time, Charles had slowly brought his blood chemistry and vital signs to what physicians believed were the best possible levels. Imagine both Charles' and his doctors' astonishment when Charles' total cholesterol suddenly dropped from 206 to 169! In addition, his LDL cholesterol level dropped from 130 to 98, his triglycerides dropped from 69 to 63, and his uric acid dropped from 2.4 to 1.2. The only change in

Charles' life was his consumption of *Rhododendron caucasicum* extract, which he had begun taking three months prior. And Charles also had proof: copies of every physical performed on him (two or three per year) since 1986.

Over time, along with Ed and Charles' reports, I received countless unsolicited letters and calls of thanks from other people throughout the United States and Canada who had realized *Rhododendron caucasicum* extract's benefits. Dozens reported drops in cholesterol levels. Heart patients reported significant reductions in chest pain and improvements in energy. People with low blood pressure reported that their blood pressures increased, while people with high blood pressure reported that their blood pressure decreased. Arthritis sufferers reported less pain and improved mobility. Many people with hemorrhoids reported reductions in or the elimination of swelling and/or bleeding. And some people with spider veins in their legs and ankles reported that the veins were decreasing in size. "They're just melting away," one letter writer said.

Dave Deslauriers in Minnesota said he had suffered from untreatable gout in one of his big toes for more than two years. He had been walking on the side of his foot ever since. But after taking *Rhododendron caucasicum* extract for just a few days, his gout disappeared.

Then came the calls from celebrities. *Rhododendron caucasicum* extract helped them "think more clearly," "move better," or "pitch better." Also, other users continued to report their problems with acid reflux were diminishing, for one thing, and their yeast problems had lessened. Others experienced fewer and less severe cold and flu episodes.

From this feedback, I know that *Rhododendron caucasicum* extract has produced the same results in Americans and Canadians as has been described in Soviet, Russian and

Georgian scientific literature. It is obvious that *Rhododendron caucasicum* extract truly is both a protector of health and a substance that heals and repairs.

I've received countless other positive reports from consumers who use Caucasian blueberry leaves extract, Georgian pomegranate ellagic acid extract, and *Rhodiola rosea* extract. These also confirm the tremendous protective and healing efficacies of these plants. And I even know about these efficacies for myself. After I started using Caucasian blueberry leaves extract, for instance, my fasting blood glucose level dropped dramatically. From 112, it now hovers between 88 and 84—normal levels. In addition, the second North American to use this extract, a diabetic who is a radio program producer, saw his blood glucose level drop by more than 30 points in three weeks.

Clearly, then, all of the plants described in this book have the power to significantly improve people's well being.

Additional Benefits

At this point, it is important to note that, while many of the most prominent health benefits produced by *Rhododendron caucasicum* extract, Georgian blueberry leaves extract, Georgian pomegranate ellagic acid extract, and *Rhodiola rosea* extract are listed in this book, many additional benefits these substances produce were not detailed for reasons of clarity, focus, and space. Also, throughout the book you may have noticed that a health benefit resulting from one substance may be similar to another substance's benefits. These sometimes overlapping benefits are due to either similar or different phytochemical activities. The great thing is, these benefits are often enhanced when two or more of the substances are used together. They provide stunning evidence of the power of these unique, beneficial, and nutrient-dense substances that have been regularly consumed by the healthiest and longest living Georgians.

Safety and Efficacy of Georgian Phytomedicines

There are thousands of nutritional products on the market in the United States today. Some are high quality, some are low quality. Some produce significant results, while some produce desired results along with potentially harmful side effects. However, it has been my experience, as well as that of several prominent scientists, product analysts, and physicians of all disciplines, that these Georgian longevity phytomedicines, *Rhododendron caucasicum* extract, Caucasian blueberry leaves extract, Georgian pomegranate ellagic acid extract, and *Rhodiola rosea* extract, are safe and effective protectors and promoters of good health and longevity.

As noted elsewhere, each of these four longevity phytomedicines has been consumed by humans, as part of a normal diet, for thousands of years. Each has been used in folk medicine by one of the longest living societies on earth for at least six hundred years to thousands of years. Each has been the subject of published laboratory and clinical research. And extracts of three of the four have been available over the counter and prescribed by medical doctors for as long as fifty years. So despite the fact that these substances are not commonly known in the West, their usefulness and safety have been confirmed again and again by scientists, physicians and lay people alike.

Common Questions

Though every effort has been made to provide all pertinent information about these extracts, there are a few questions that remain to be answered. For instance, some readers may be wondering what they will feel after consuming the extracts—whether they will immediately notice a difference in their health. Others may wonder why they haven't heard about these plants until now. Still others will question why all Russians aren't consuming these plant extracts, and why Western pharmaceutical firms haven't produced drugs or other products from the plants. All are reasonable questions, and all are answered below.

ARE THE BENEFITS ALWAYS NOTICEABLE?

The answer to that question is that some of these plant extracts' benefits are noticeable, and some are not.

Benefits that will likely go unnoticed will be those related to so-called "silent" longer-term diseases. The fact is that because we normally are not aware of free radical damage, and the onset and early progression of aging-related disorders such as cancers, atherosclerosis, arteriosclerosis, brain degeneration, etc., we would not know when the onset and early progression of these conditions are inhibited. Nonetheless, we can see from major published studies that all of these Georgian plants extracts and/or their primary constituents do, in fact, inhibit free radical damage and slow the onset and progression of certain cancers, heart disease, brain degeneration, and other ills. In using the extracts to prevent and treat these diseases, we can trust scientific research that the extracts are, in fact, having the effect we desire.

With other disorders, people will likely notice the benefits, however. For example, people who know their blood pressure and blood chemistry (i.e., glucose, cholesterol, triglycerides, and uric acid levels) prior to using these Georgian plant extracts will be able to see improvements in future test results. However, they should note that it sometimes takes a few weeks of use before the extracts' effects are manifest. Beyond the tests, those with disorders who have very noticeable symptoms will be most likely to discern the extracts' results. Some of these disorders include obesity, capillary fragility (which visibly manifests itself as varicose veins, spider veins, hemorrhoids, bloody noses, bleeding gums, and broken capillaries of the eyes and face), angina, mitral valve prolapse, arthritis, gout, bacterial and viral infections, some sugar imbalances, and depression and stress disorders.

Other noticeable effects include improvements in mental and physical performance. So, in other words, following the regular use of a relevant Georgian antiaging plant extract, a person who suffers from angina should experience less frequent and less severe chest pain. A person who suffers from arthritis should experience less pain and greater range of motion. And a person who suffers from two or three severe colds per year should notice a decrease in both the frequency and severity of colds.

WHY HAVEN'T WE HEARD ABOUT THIS BEFORE?

The tremendous contributions of Georgian researchers were almost always unknown by Westerners due to the political and scientific isolation of the Georgian republic, formerly part of the Soviet Union. It must be remembered that the Soviet Union was a closed society, and relations between that country and the West were strained. In addition, the few examples of Soviet scientific research that were allowed to be released to the world were seldom reviewed by nongovernmental Western scientists, because few Western scientists had the ability or took the time to read Russian. (And almost no one can read Georgian other than the Georgians.) Moreover, translations are time consuming and cost prohibitive, especially for academics and publishers that usually operate under tight budgets. Also, for years, it has been difficult enough for Western scientists to process the glut of research produced in the West alone. Unfortunately, researchers in the West did little if any research on the substances presented in this book until recently.

Things changed tremendously with the fall of the Iron Curtain, and with simultaneous and continuous improvements in communications. Today, scientists of the former Soviet bloc countries are exchanging ideas with the rest of the free world at an ever increasing rate. Because of these countries' liberation and our growing world consciousness, we are now able to present the beneficial research—performed by serious, world-class scientists—that has been unavailable to us until now.

Keep in mind that the Russian and Georgian scientists who performed their studies did so without any expectation of outside recognition or monetary gain. They devoted their lives to discovering substances that could benefit humanity, and most have had to wait a long time to share their results with the world.

WHY HAVEN'T ALL RUSSIANS UTILIZED THESE SUBSTANCES?

Although southern Russia borders Georgia, the lifestyles of Russians and Georgians are and have always been very different. They are, after all, two unique countries and cultures. For example, the general Russian diet has historically been quite poor. It was primarily composed of only a few foods, such as potatoes, cabbage, and bread.[1,2] Contrast that with the myriad foods contained in the traditional Georgian diet, and the differences become quite clear.

In addition, although Russian and Georgian research produced a wealth of scientific discoveries, few of these evolved into readily available products in Russia. This was due to the lack of a market economy and all that it entails—private ownership, entrepreneurship, venture capital, noncentralized planning, production, packaging, distribution, retailing, marketing and advertising, fulfillment transportation, and, of course, the incomes people can earn through capitalism to buy the products they desire. It's certainly difficult to use a substance if you can't afford to buy it, and if your country's market system can't support its production and distribution.

In contrast, until recently Georgians have always been surrounded by the lush bounty of super-nutrition described herein. It was simply a part of their traditional culture. Furthermore, the Georgians who made health-benefiting discoveries almost always put them to immediate use for their fellow Georgians. Their country's distinctive, healthful *modus vivendi*, including the fraternal sharing of science and life, has been known for years throughout the former Soviet republics as Georgian style.[3]

WHERE ARE THE PHARMACEUTICAL FIRMS?

It takes approximately fifteen years and costs between $100 million and $500 million to win approval for a drug to be developed and marketed for specific use(s) in the United States.[4,5] The only way a pharmaceutical company can recoup such huge expenses and make a profit is by obtaining a patent, which gives the company the sole right to sell a formulation for specific use(s).[4] However, a substance or a formula cannot be patented in the United States for a specific use, if it were publically used anywhere in the world for the same purpose more than one year prior to the date of patent.[6]

The substances described in this book are gifts of nature that have been used by the public for hundreds, and in some cases thousands, of years. Moreover, as mentioned, although each substance presented in this book is primarily known for a specific use, each also has several additional known efficacies for which it has also been used. Therefore, acquiring a patent on any of these substances, or any derivatives thereof, for any of the purposes described herein would be nearly impossible. Because of these factors, pharmaceutical firms must, from a business standpoint, neglect most previously used natural health substances and instead attempt to develop alternative drugs for which they can secure exclusive rights through patent ownership.

Nonetheless, there are reports of pharmaceutical firms currently attempting to develop synthetic analogs of some of the substances described here. If they win approval for their formulations, these pharmaceutical firms will likely heavily promote them to physicians, who will prescribe the formulations to their patients.

Healthy Longevity

At some point, almost everyone thinks about how much more he or she could accomplish with a little more time. Unfortunately, by the time most people reach their apexes of composure, experience, kindness, knowledge, and wisdom, their bodies have begun to noticeably break down and slow down. The mind soon follows. So imagine what a wonderful gift it would be to our families, to ourselves, and to society if we could add even a few more healthy years to our lives. Imagine the good that could be done.

Most scientists believe that humans are quite capable of living in good health well into their 120s and beyond. The only things stopping such extended healthy longevity are cellular damage and aging-related illnesses. In fact, almost all illnesses, other than those caused by infections, injuries, and genetic defects, are related to aging. Almost all aging-related illnesses are caused by cellular damage. And the vast majority of cellular damage is caused by oxidation/free radicals. But because our physiological systems can't repair the oxidative/free radical damage as quickly as it occurs, we age.

Until genetic engineering is mastered, the best way to slow the clock on aging is by maintaining a low-calorie and low-carbohydrate, nutritious dietary lifestyle, by engaging in low-impact exercise, and by consuming an array of superpowerful antioxidants/free radical neutralizers. These three factors slow the onset and progression of aging-related diseases, which results in less stress on all systems and which allows us to live in good health longer. In other words, to live longer and healthier lives, we need to live the commonsense lifestyle of traditional Georgians.

Today, the four Georgian plant medicines described in this book are available as potent, standardized extracts to the North American public. Each of the plant extracts, *Rhododendron caucasicum* extract, Caucasian blueberry leaves extract, Georgian pomegranate ellagic acid extract, and *Rhodiola rosea* extract, contains unique, natural blends of superpowerful antioxidants/free radical neutralizers. The extracts' efficacies are both specific and wide-ranging. And each plant has successfully been used to prevent and treat illnesses for hundreds of years. Their efficacies have been demonstrated by studies conducted at many of the world's leading scientific research institutions. So truly, the answer to how to live longer lives is staring us in the face.

The desire to slow the clock on aging is a noble one. The sooner one converts desire to action, the better.

Quick Reference

Rhododendron Caucasicum Extract

KEY CONSTITUENTS

Chlorogenic acid, gallic acid, rhododendrons, salidroside, tyrosol, hydroxycinnamic acid derivatives, taxifolin+astilbin (taxifolins), quercitrin, quercetin and quercetin-glycosides, kaempherol, myrecetin, rutin, isoramnithin, arbutin, proanthocyanidins and anthocyanins (cyanidin, delphinidin, petunidin, malvidin), (-)-epicatechin, (-)-epicatechingallate, (+)-gallocatechin, (-)-epicatechin.

PRIMARY ACTIVITIES

- Acts as a powerful antioxidant/free radical neutralizer
- Helps the body adapt to stresses caused by physical, chemical, and biological factors

- Reduces fat absorption
- Breaks up fat from fat storage tissue and makes it available to be burned off during exercise
- Strengthens blood vessels and helps prevent the following: strokes in which the blood vessels of the brain become weak and burst; varicose veins; hemorrhoids; bloody noses; bleeding gums; broken capillaries of the eye, face, and body
- Reduces LDL (bad) cholesterol levels
- Protects cholesterol from free radical damage
- Helps normalize blood pressures
- Helps normalize pulse
- Improves blood circulation in the heart
- Reduces chest pain/angina
- Helps prevent and treat heart disease
- Reduces the production of hyaluronidase, which is a cause of colon cancer and may be a root cause of arthritis
- Reduces arthritic pain and increases mobility
- Reduces muscle pain, especially in the face and eyes
- Lowers uric acid, thereby preventing and treating gout
- Detoxifies the liver
- Helps prevent glaucoma and improves vision
- Kills several species of pathogenic (bad) bacteria
- Decreases the frequency and severity of colds and flu
- Limits DNA damage caused by carcinogens

RECOMMENDED USE

Take between 50 milligrams and 100 milligrams two to three times per day before meals. *Rhododendron caucasicum* extract is very powerful. Therefore, first-time users should start by taking a low dosage.

Caucasian Blueberry Leaves Extract

KEY CONSTITUENTS

Chlorogenic acid, neochlorogenic acid, 4-caffeoylquinic acid, 3-coumaroylqunic acid, hydroxycinnamic acid, coumaric acid, salidroside, tyrosol, ericolin, myricetin, arbutin, anthocyanosides, quercetin, rutin.

PRIMARY ACTIVITIES

- Acts as a powerful antioxidant/free radical neutralizer
- Reduces sugar absorption
- Reduces glucose production by the liver
- Reduces blood glucose levels
- Helps maintain balanced glucose levels
- Helps prevent and treat diabetes
- Reduces LDL (bad) cholesterol levels
- Protects cholesterol from free radical damage
- Reduces triglyceride levels
- Helps prevent and treat cardiovascular diseases
- Inhibits peroxynitrite, a cause of heart inflammation and brain degeneration
- Inhibits the enzyme 5-lipoxygenase, which causes inflammation and brain degeneration
- Helps protect against brain-degenerative diseases, such as Parkinson's disease
- Inhibits the effects of cancer-causing nitrites found in tobacco products, cured meats, fried foods, baked goods, cereals, and vegetables
- Treats gastric colitis
- Reduces pesticide damage
- Reduces radiation damage

- Limits DNA damage caused by carcinogens
- Kills some species of pathogenic (bad) bacteria
- Decreases the frequency and severity of colds and flu
- Inhibits herpes simplex viruses Types 1 and 2
- Inhibits HIV

RECOMMENDED USE

Take between 150 milligrams and 300 milligrams (although many people take 400 milligrams) three times per day about 15 minutes before meals. Caucasian blueberry leaves extract is very powerful and will lower blood glucose levels. Therefore, diabetics and others with glucose imbalances should carefully monitor their blood glucose levels and adjust their diets and the medications they are taking accordingly.

Georgian Pomegranate/Ellagic Acid Extract

KEY CONSTITUENTS

Ellagic acid and anthocyanidins: cyanidin, delphinidin 3-glucoside, delphinidin 3,5-glucoside, cyanidin 3-glucoside, cyanidin 3,5-diglucoside, cyanidin 3-glucose, pelargonidin, delphinidin.

PRIMARY ACTIVITIES

- Acts as a powerful antioxidant/free radical neutralizer
- Limits DNA damage caused by carcinogens
- Kills cancer cells
- Inhibits the multiplication of cancer cells
- Inhibits metastasizing (spreading) of cancer cells

- Protects against alcohol-induced damage to the stomach and intestines
- Reduces the aggregation and retention (clustering) of LDL (bad) cholesterol in the bloodstream
- Protects LDL (bad) cholesterol and HDL (good) cholesterol from free radical damage
- Reduces high blood pressure
- Relaxes the blood vessels
- Inhibits certain inflammatory processes
- Helps prevent and treat atherosclerosis
- Destroys certain intestinal worms
- Helps protect the blood, kidneys, and liver from environmental pollutants
- Inhibits several species of pathogenic (bad) bacteria

RECOMMENDED USE

Take at least 50 milligrams two or three times per day.

Rhodiola Rosea Extract

KEY CONSTITUENTS

Rosavin, rosin, rosarin, salidroside (rhodioloside), tyrosol, rodiolin, rodionin, rodiosin, acetylrodalgin, tricin, rosiridol, rosaridin, daucosterol, beta-sitosterol, chlorogenic acid, hydroxycinnamic acid, gallic acid.

PRIMARY ACTIVITIES

- Acts as a powerful antioxidant/free radical neutralizer

- Helps the body adapt to stresses caused by physical, chemical, and biological factors
- Helps prevent and treat depression
- Lessens the severity of side effects caused by tricyclic antidepressants
- Helps prevent and treat stress disorders
- Helps prevent and treat neuroses
- Reduces afternoon sluggishness
- Improves mood and attitude
- Helps regulate sleep
- Reduces the severity and pain of illnesses by reducing the stress associated with illnesses
- Improves intellectual work performance
- Improves physical work performance
- Improves resistance to high-altitude sickness
- Builds bulk muscle when used by body builders without steroid-like side effects
- Breaks up fat from fat storage tissue and makes it available to be burned off during exercise
- Decreases recovery times following intellectual and physical performances
- Improves memory
- Improves hearing
- Protects against stress-induced heart damage
- Prevents heart arrhythmias
- Helps regulate blood pressure, pulse, and blood circulation
- Inhibits tumor growth
- Inhibits metastasizing (spreading) of cancer cells
- Decreases the side effects of certain anticancer drugs
- Improves male sexual performance
- Helps regulate menstrual cycles

SAFETY CONCERNS

The species *Rhodiola rosea* has been found to be safe and nonaddicting for both animals and humans.[1] However, Richard P. Brown, M.D., Patricia L. Gerbarg, M.D., and Zakir Ramazanov, Ph.D., state that "*Rhodiola rosea* has an active antidepressant effect, [and] it should not be used in individuals with bipolar disorder, who are vulnerable to becoming manic when give antidepressants or stimulants."[1]

RECOMMENDED USE

Take between 50 milligrams and 200 milligrams one to three times per day. *Rhodiola rosea* is best absorbed if taken approximately thirty minutes before meals or two hours after meals. (Based upon *Rhodiola rosea* standardized to 3 percent rosavin and 0.8 percent to 1 percent salidroside. Adjust dosages according to different concentrations of rosavin and salidroside.)

Generalized Explanation of Georgian Extraction Methods

**Rhododendron caucasicum spring leaves
Caucasian blueberry spring leaves
Georgian pomegranate whole fruit
Rhodiola rosea root**

• The desired plant material is selected, picked, bagged, and delivered to the extraction facility. The plant material is washed and then loaded onto conveyors which deliver it into dryer units.

• Following drying, the plant material is ground into a powder.

• The dried, ground plant material is processed with solutions which extract nutrients.

• The resulting fluid extract is then filtered and centrifuged until the extracts' content of key nutrients has been standardized to optimum levels:

- *Rhododendron caucasicum* extract
- (40% polyphenolics, 5% taxifolins.)
- Caucasian blueberry leaves extract
- (20% chlorogenic and hydroxycinnamic acids.)
- Georgian pomegranate ellagic acid extract
- (70% polyphenolics, 40% ellagic acid.)
- *Rhodiola rosea* extract
- (3% rosavins, 0.8% salidroside.)

- The standardized, concentrated liquid extract is spray dried back into a powder.

- Samples of the dried extract powder are assayed to confirm their contents of polyphenolics and specific phenolics, and are tested to confirm compliance with all Food Grade Standards.

- The dried extract is loaded into 25-gallon drums, and technicians seal the drums. The sealed drums of extract, along with a Certificate of Analysis, are shipped to the United States via air freight. Upon arrival, U.S. Customs agents examine the shipment and the Certificate of Analysis, and provide a Customs Clearance Certificate. U.S. Food and Drug Administration personnel examine the shipment, and provide F.D.A. Certification. The drums of extract then are shipped to a secure, temperature- and humidity-controlled warehouse/lab facility. The shipment and the Certificate of Analysis are re-examined by U.S. technicians. The drums of extract are then shipped to encapsulation and bottling companies as ordered.

Generalized Explanation of Encapsulation and Bottling

- Upon arrival at an encapsulation and bottling facility, the extract is examined to confirm that it complies with the data reported on the Certificate of Analysis. Following confirmation of integrity, the extract then moves onto formulation.

- If the extract is to be part of a formulation, which includes additional nutrients, the other nutrients are added. The final formulation is placed into equipment, which mixes the formulation until correct amounts of each nutrient will be found in each capsule or tablet to be produced.

- Samples of the final mixed formulation are analyzed to determine "stickiness" and "ease of flow" through encapsulation equipment. The encapsulation equipment is calibrated accordingly.

- The formulation then is deposited into sterile stainless steel holding cells. From there, the formulation is fed into either an encapsulation machine, which encapsulates an exact amount of the formula within each capsule, or into a tabulating machine, which forms the formula into tablets.

- The capsules or tablets then are transferred into bottling equipment, which deposits a set amount of capsules or tablets into individual bottles, seals the bottles, labels the bottles and deposits the bottles into shipping boxes.

- The end product is then shipped to wholesalers, distributors, retailers, and consumers as ordered.

Endnotes

INTRODUCTION

1. Smith T. J. 1999. In Renewal: The Anti-Aging Revolution. New York. St. Martins Paperbacks. P. 315-338
2. Pfizer. 2002. Opening nature's medicine cabinet: the science of medicine. Pfizer, Inc. http://www.pfizer.com/science/openingnaturefrm.html
3. Myatt R. G. 1997. Plant. The Grolier Multimedia Encyclopedia. Grolier Interactive, Inc.
4. Davidson M. W. and Florida State University. 2002. The phytochemical collection. http://micro.magnet.fsu.edu/phytochemicals
5. Ramazanov Z. 1997, 2001, 2002, 2003. Telephone interviews of Zakır Ramazanov, Ph.D., by the author, Shaffer Fox
6. Barclay L. 2002. A tasty alternative to vitamins. http://www.parsonline.com/articles1.htm
7. UIHC (University of Iowa Health Care). 2001. Medical museum. Nature's pharmacy: ancient knowledge, modern medicine. http://www.unihealthcare.com/depts/medmuseum/galleryexhibits/nature-spharmacy.html7.
8. Asami D. K., Hong Y-J, Barrett D. M., Mitchell A. E. 2003. Comparison of the total phenolic and ascorbic acid content of freeze-dried and air-dried marionberry, strawberry, and corn grown using conventional, organic, and sustainable agricultural practices. Journal of Agricultural and Food Chemistry. 51: 1237-1241.
9. Lee C. L. 1997. Soviet Education. The Grolier Multimedia Encyclopedia. Grolier Interactive, Inc.

10. Turkevich J. 1997. Chromatography. The Grolier Multimedia Encyclopedia. Grolier Interactive, Inc.
11. Graham L. R. 1989. Russian & Soviet Science and Technology. History of Science Society Newsletter. 18(4): Supplement.
12. Cross J. L. 1995. A Guide to the Russian Academy of Sciences. Austin, TX. Cross Associates. 1st Edition. Pp. 11, 14.

CHAPTER 1. GEORGIA AND GEORGIAN LONGEVITY

1. WABF (The World Almanac Book of Facts). 1998. Mountains: Caucasus (Europe-Asia). Mahway, New Jersey. World Almanac Books. P. 591.
2. GEF PDF-A. 2001. Recovery, Conservation, and Sustainable Use of Georgia's Agrobiodiversity.
3. BISNIS (Business Information Service for the Newly Independent States). 2004. Republic of Georgia Commercial Overview. http://www.bisnis.doc.gov/bis-nis/country/9906gacomov.htm
4. GIZO. 2002. Georgia. http://www.skategoal.com/gizo_org/gizo.htm
5. Reuffler M. 2002. A Psychopolitical Action Project, Healing A Collective, The Village of Bakuriani, Republic of Georgia, 1994-1997. Association for the Advancement of Psychosynthesis. http://www.aap-psychosynthesis.org/collective.html
6. Benet S. 1976. In How to live to be 100. The life-style of the people of the Caucasus. Pp. 23. New York. The Dial Press.
7. Mchedishvili D. 1999. Georgian language: The history of written language. http://members.tripod.com/ggdavid/georgia/language/bookhist.htm
8. Kaplan R. D. 2000. Where Europe Vanishes. The Atlantic Monthly. November.
9. Ethnologue: Languages of the World. Languages of Georgia. http://www.ethnologue.com/show_country.asp?name=Georgia.
10. USDS (U. S. & Foreign Commercial Service and the U. S. Department of State). 1998. Travel and Tourism Services. http://www.tradeport.org/ts/countries/georgia/isa/isar0001.html
11. Gabunia L., Vekua A., Lordkipanidze D., Swisher C. C. III., Ferring R., Justus A., Nioradze M., Tvalchrelidze M., Anton S. C., Bosinski G., Joris O., Lumley M. A., Majsuradze G., Mouskhelishvili A. 2000. Earliest Pleistocene hominid cranial remains from Dmanisi, Republic of Georgia: taxonomy, geological setting, and age. Science. May 12;288(5468):1019-25.
12. Gugliotta. 2000. Out of Africa, an early migration. Eurasian skulls point to human forebears on go. Washington Post. May 12. P. A03.
13. O'Hara V. 2001. Funds pay off at Dmanisi: Fossils provide new evidence of hominid migration. http://www.leakeyfoundation.org/anthroquest_2001_04.html14.
14. Schaffner R. 2000. Science headlines Thursday May 11, 2000. Early human migrants' fossils found by Paul Recer, AP science writer. Associated Press; Creature Chronicles. http://www.n2.net/prey/bigfoot/hominids/earlyhumans.htm5.
15. Anton S. 2001. Telephone interview of Susan Anton, Ph.D., by the author, Shaffer Fox. September 7, 2003.

16. Vekua A., Lordkipanidze D., Rightmire G. P., Agusti J., Ferring R., Maisuradze G., Mouskhelishvili A., Nioradze M., Ponce de Leon M., Tappen M., Tvalchrelidze M., Zollikofer C. 2002. A new skull of early homo from Dmanisi, Georgia. Science. July 5. 297:85-89.

17. Gore R. 2002. New find. National Geographic. August. Cover story.

18. Szuromi P. 2002. More from Dmanisi. This Week in Science. Science. July 5.

19. Mchedishvili D. 1999. History of Georgia. http://members.tripod.com/ggdavid/georgia/history.htm

20. Lydolph P. E. 1964. In Geography of the U. S. S. R. P. 152. New York. John Wiley and Sons, Inc.

21. Temple (The Temple). 2000. The Temple. P.10-15. Tblisi. Tblisi State University Press.

22. Rosen R. 1999. In Georgia. A sovereign country of the Caucasus. Hong Kong, China. Odyssey Publications Ltd. Pp. 81-82.

23. Lordkipanidze D. 2002. Telephone interview of Professor David Lordkipanidze, Ph.D., Deputy Director of the Georgian State Museum, by the author, Shaffer Fox. June 17.

24. Fornara C. W. 1997. Greece, ancient. The Grolier Multimedia Encyclopedia. Grolier Interactive, Inc.

25. Anchabadze G. 2002. History of Georgia. http://www.parliament.ge/GENERAL/HISTORY/his1.html

26. Metreveli R. 2002. Brief History of Georgia. http://www.members.tripod.com/amik78/GeorgiaHistory.htm

27. Goldstein D. 1999. In The Georgian feast: the vibrant culture and savory food of the Republic of Georgia. Los Angeles. University of California Press. P. xiv.

28. Benet S. 1976. In How to live to be 100. The life-style of the people of the Caucasus. P. 22. New York. The Dial Press.

29. Benet S. 1976. In How to live to be 100. The life-style of the people of the Caucasus. Pp. 79-80. New York. The Dial Press.

30. Kemertelidze E. 2003. History of the Institute of Pharmacochemistry of the Georgian Academy of Sciences.

31. Benet S. 1976. In How to live to be 100. The life-style of the people of the Caucasus. P. 91. New York. The Dial Press.

32. Ramazanov Z. 1997, 2001, 2002, 2003. Telephone interviews of Zakir Ramazanov, Ph.D., by the author, Shaffer Fox.

33. Lelashvili N. and Dalakishvili S. 1984. Genetic study of high longevity index populations. Mechanisms of Ageing and Development. 28(2-3):261-71.

34. BPS (The Berkeley Program in Soviet and Post-Soviet Studies.. 1997. Institutions, Identity, and Ethnic Conflict: International Experience and Its Implications for the Caucasus. Conference report. Berkeley Program in Soviet and Post-Soviet Studies, Center for Slavic and East European Studies, Institute of International Studies. http://socrates.berkeley.edu/~bsp/publications/1997_01-conf.pdf

35. Pond E. 1988. In From the Yaroslavsky Station: Russia Perceived. P. 116. New York. Universe Books.

36. Raef M. 1997. Russia, History of. The Grolier Multimedia Encyclopedia. Grolier Interactive, Inc.

37. Hewitt B. G. 1995. Georgia: Contemporary life and politics. Main population of Georgia (1979 & 1989). http://www.abkhazia.org/georgia.html

38. Rosen R. 1999. In Georgia. A Sovereign Country of the Caucasus. Hong Kong, China. Odyssey Publications Ltd. P. 30.
39. Labbate G. 2002. Languages Spoken in Georgia. Statistics included in written response to the author, Shaffer Fox, by Gabriel Labbate, Ph.D., sub-regional project advisor to the GEF, and team leader of the National Human Development Report, Georgia, reporting Republic of Georgia State Department of Statistics and Georgian Population Census figures for 1989, and results of reviews and analysis of statistics by Georgian academicians.
40. OPG. (Orthodox Patriarchate of Georgia). 2002. Welcome to Orthodox Georgia: Education. http://www.orthodox-patriarchate-of-georgia.org.ge/Pilgrimage/Pilgrim.htm
41. Bronfenbrenner U. 1972. In Two worlds of childhood U. S. and U. S. S. R. New York. Touchstone edition. Simon and Schuster.
42. Fischer J. 1972. In Two worlds of childhood U. S. and U. S. S. R. by Urie Bronfenbrenner. Cover commentary. New York. Touchstone edition. Simon and Schuster.
43. GA. 1996. Republic of Georgia: Policy framework paper, 1996-1998. Prepared by Georgian authorities in collaboration with the staffs of the International Monetary Fund and the World Bank. 3. Education; 53. February 9.
44. DIS (The Danish Immigration Service). 2002. 5.0. Language Act. http://www.udlst.dk/sjle1/georgien99/kap5.html
45. Suny R. G. 1997. Institutions, Identity, and Ethnic Conflict: International Experience and Its Implications for the Caucasus. Conference report. Fragments and Forms: National and Supernational Identities in Georgia. P. 67. Berkeley Program in Soviet and Post-Soviet Studies, Center for Slavic and East European Studies, Institute of International Studies. http://socrates.berkeley.edu/~bsp/publications/1997_01-conf.pdf
46. Hinton L. 1997. Institutions, Identity, and Ethnic Conflict: International Experience and Its Implications for the Caucasus. Conference report. Institutional Protections for Endangered Languages. P. 7. Berkeley Program in Soviet and Post-Soviet Studies, Center for Slavic and East European Studies, Institute of International Studies. http://socrates.berkeley.edu/~bsp/publications/1997_01-conf.pdf
47. GAUSA (Georgian Association in the United States of America, Inc.). 2002. Georgian history and culture. http://www.georgianassociation.org/culture.htm
48. TPT (Tbilisipastimes). 2002. Languages. http://www.tbilisipastimes.com/language.html
49. IFES (International Fellowship of Evangelical Students) 2002. IFES Year Teams: Caucasus Republics, Georgia & Armenia. Http://www.ifesworld.org/teams/countryprofiles/caucasus.htm
50. Snowdon D. A., Ostwald S. K., Kane R. L. 1989. Education, survival, and independence in elderly Catholic sisters 1936-1988. American Journal of Epidemiology. November;130(5):999-1012.
51. Snowdon D. A., Kemper S. J., Mortimer J. A., Greiner L. H., Wekstein D. R., Markesbery W. R. 1996. Linguistic ability in early life and cognitive function and Alzheimer's disease in late life. Findings from the Nun Study. Journal of the American Medical Association. February 21;275(7):528-32.
52. Snowdon D. A., Greiner L. H., Kemper S. J., Nanayakkara N., Mortimer J. A.

1999. In Linguistic Ability in Early Life and Longevity: Findings from the Nun Study. The Paradoxes of Longevity. Pp. 103-113. New York. Springer-Verlag New York, Inc.

53. Snowdon D. A., Geeiner L. H., Markesbery W. R. 2000. Linguistic ability in early life and the neuropathology of Alzheimer's disease and cerebrovascular disease. Findings from the Nun Study. Annals of the New York Academy of Sciences. April; 903:34-8.

54. Benet S. 1976. In How to live to be 100. The life-style of the people of the Caucasus. Pp. 49-50. New York. The Dial Press.

55. Benet S. 1976. In How to live to be 100. The life-style of the people of the Caucasus. P. 7. New York. The Dial Press.

56. Closter L. 2002. World Religions and Cultures. http://wrc.lingnet.org/default.htm

57. Ibrevise. 2002. Stalin Page 2. http://www.geocities.com/ibrevise/stalin2.html

58. Von Lilienfeld F. 2002. Reflections on the Current State of the Georgian Church and Nation. http://www.anglefire.com/ga/Georgian/history.html

59. Anchabadze G. 2002a. Georgia in 1921-1945. http://www.parliament.ge/GENERAL HISTORY/his12.html

60. Tarkhan-Mouravi G. 1997. 70 Years of Soviet Georgia. http://rolfgross.tripod.com/Texts/Giahistory.htm

61. DSG (Department of Statistics, Republic of Georgia). 2002. Population 100 years and older. Provided by Merab Pachulia

62. CDG (Census Department of Georgia). 2002a. Census data & survey data: 100+ population. November 18.

63. CDG (Census Department of Georgia). 2002b. Population in the thousands for the years 1926, 2000, 2001, 2002. November 28.

64. CIA (Central Intelligence Agency). 1994. Georgia. http://www.departments. Bucknell.edu/russian/facts/georgia.html

65. WWA (Reader's Digest Wide World Atlas). 1979. Pleasantville, NY.

66. MBG (Missouri Botanical Garden). 2002a. Rare, Endangered and Vulnerable Plants of the Republic of Georgia. http://www.mobot.org/MOBOT/Research/georgia/introduction.shtml

67. Pacholia, M. 2002. Telephone interview of Merab Pacholia in Tblisi, Georgia, by the author, Shaffer Fox. April 10.

68. GH (Georgia). 1994. Health. http://lcweb2.loc.gov/cgi-bin/query/r?frd/cstdy:@field(DOCID+ge0045

69. Benet S. 1976. In How to live to be 100. The life-style of the people of the Caucasus. P. 82-83. New York. The Dial Press.

70. Benet S. 1976. In How to live to be 100. The life-style of the people of the Caucasus. P. 104. New York. The Dial Press.

71. Kant A. K. 2000. Consumption of energy-dense, nutrient-poor foods by adult Americans: nutritional and health implications. The third National Health and Nutrition Examination Survey, 1988-1994. American Journal of Clinical Nutrition. October;72(4):929-36.

72. GORBI (Georgian Opinion Research Business International). 2000. Lifestyle Georgia 2000. http://www.gorbi.com

73. LC (Library of Congress). 1994. Georgia. http://lcweb2.loc.gov/cgi-bin/query/r?frd/cstdy:@field(DOCID+ge0036)

74. ASH (Action on Smoking and Health) 2001. Fact Sheet Number 21: Tobacco in

the Developing World. September.
http://www.ash.org.uk/html/factsheets/html/fact21.html
75. GAP (Georgia Parliament). 2002. Privatization. http://www.parliament.ge/ECO-
NOMICS/PRIVAT.htm
76. GCIS (Georgia Consular Information Sheet). 2001. Medical Facilities.
http://travel.state.gov/georgia.html. November 28.

CHAPTER 2: THE GEORGIAN DIET

1.Benet S. 1976. In How to live to be 100. The life-style of the people of the
Caucasus. P. 91. New York. The Dial Press.
2. Ramazanov Z. 1997, 2000, 2001, 2002. Telephone interviews of Zakir
Ramazanov, Ph.D., by the author, Shaffer Fox.
3. Benet S. 1976. In How to live to be 100. The life-style of the people of the
Caucasus. P. 94. New York. The Dial Press.
4. Rosen R. 1999. In Georgia. A sovereign country of the Caucasus. Hong Kong,
China. Odyssey Publications Ltd. P. 85.
5. Lopez-Jimenez F., Mittleman M., Maclure M., Tofler G., Sherwood J., Muller J.
2000. Heavy meals could trigger heart attacks. Veterans Administration
Research and Development. Presentation to the American Heart Association
scientific meeting in New Orleans. Nov. 14.
6. Finkel E. 2003. The Science of Aging.
http://www.wehi.edu.au/resources/vce_biol_science/articles/fonkel5.html
7. Butler R. N. 2002. Written testimony of Robert N. Butler, M. D., before the
Senate Special Committee on Aging. Baton Rouge, Louisiana. August 15.
8. PM (PubMed). 2001. Keyword searches: Harman D.; Weindruch R. National
Center for Biotechnology Information, National Library of Medicine, National
Institutes of Health. http://www.ncbi.nlm.nih.gov/entrez/query
9. PM (PubMed). 2001. Keyword searches: Calorie restriction. National Center for
Biotechnology Information, National Library of Medicine, National Institutes
of Health. http://www.ncbi.nlm.nih.gov/entrez/query
10. Weindruch and Walford. 1982. Dietary restriction in mice beginning at 1 year of
age: effect on life-span and spontaneous cancer incidence. Science. Mar
12;215(4538):415-8.
11. Lam M. and Sulindro M. 2001. Calories that count.
http://www.a3r.org/briefs/calories_that_count.cfm
12. Ramsey J. J., Colman R. J., Binkley N. C., Christensen J. D., Gresl T. A., Kemnit J.
W., Weindruch R. 2000. Dietary restriction and aging in rhesus monkeys: the
University of Wisconsin study. Experimental Gerontology. December;35(9-
10):1131-49.
13. Wanagat J., Allison D. B., Weindruch R. 1999. Caloric intake and aging: mechanisms in rodents and study in nonhuman primates. Toxicological Sciences: An
Official Journal of the Society of Toxicology. December;52(2Suppliment):35-
40.
14. Benet S. 1976. In How to live to be 100. The life-style of the people of the
Caucasus. P. 82-83. New York. The Dial Press.
15. Lichine A. 1981. In Alexis Lichine's new encyclopedia of wines & spirits. New
York. Alfred A. Knopf, Inc. P. 421.

16. Rosen R. 1999. In Georgia. A sovereign country of the Caucasus. Hong Kong, China. Odyssey Publications Ltd. Pp. 81-82.
17. Goldstein D. 1999. In The Georgian feast: the vibrant culture and savory food of the Republic of Georgia. Los Angeles. University of California Press. P. xiv.
18. Lordkipanidze D. 2002. Telephone interview of Professor David Lordkipanidze, Ph.D., Deputy Director of the Georgian State Museum, by the author, Shaffer Fox. June 17.
19. SAMCO (Samkharadze & Company, Ltd.). 2001. The Best Wine from Georgia: Viniculture and Winemaking in Georgia. http://travelguide.ge/georgia/article2.htm
20. IUGTG (International Union Georgian Travel Guide). 2002. Religions Change, but the Wine Remain. http://travelguide.ge/georgia/article2.htm
21. GEF PDF-A. 2001. Recovery, Conservation, and Sustainable Use of Georgia's Agrobiodiversity.
22. Sulaberidze M. 2002. Wine Sector Overview Report. http://www.cerma.ge/reports/WINE%20SECTOR%20OVERVIEW.pdf
23. Landrault N., Poucheret P., Ravel P., Gase F., Cros G., Teissedre P-L. 2001. Antioxidant capacities and phenolic levels of French wines from different varieties and vintages. Journal of Agricultural and Food Chemistry. 49:3341-3348.
24. Pellegrini N., Simonetti P., Gardana C., Brenna O., Brighenti F., Pietta P. 2000. Polyphenol content and total antioxidant activity of vini novelli (Young Red Wines). Journal of Agricultural and Food Chemistry. 48:732-735.
25. Chklukvishvili I., Ramazanov Z., Khachidze O. 2000. Comparative characteristics of some Georgia and Spanish wines according to the content of polyphenolic substances and antioxidant activity. Bulletin of the Georgian Academy of Sciences. 161, 162, 2000.
26. USDA. 2001. U. S. per capita coffee consumption. Horticultural and Tropical Products Division, FAS/USDA. http://www.ffas.usda.gov/htp/tropical/2001/06-01/coffusco.pdf
27. MSN (MadSci Network). 2001. Chemistry: What are all the ingredients in coffee? http://www.madsci.org/posts/archives/dec2001/1007419335.Ch.r.html
28. Van Dam R. M. and Feskens E. J. M. 2002. Coffee consumption and the risk of type 2 diabetes mellitus. Lancet. 360:1477-78.
29. Abidoff M. 1997. Rhododendron caucasicum: pharmacology and phytochemistry. Moscow. Center for Modern Medicine.
30. Abidoff M. & Kekelidze N. 1997. Effect of Rhododendron caucasicum herbal supplement on dietary fat absorption and weight loss in obese patients. Moscow Center for Modern Medicine. February 12.
31. Teselkin I. O., Zhambalova B. A., Babenkova I. V., Tiukavkina N. A. 1996. Antioxidant properties of dihydroquercetin. Biofizika. 41(3):620-4.
32. Prior R. L., and Cao G. 1999. Variability in dietary antioxidant related natural product supplements: the need for method of standardization. JANA Vol. 2. Pp. 46-56.
33. Closa D., Torres M., Hotter G., Bioque G., León OS., Gelpí E., Rósello-Catafau J. 1997. Prostanoids and free radicals in Cl4C-induced hepatotoxicity in rats: effect of astilbin. Prostaglandins, Leukotrienes, and Essential Fatty Acids. 56(4):331-334.
34. Rossiyski D. 1954. Rhododendron: a new remedy for regulation of blood circulation insufficiency. Pharmacology and Toxicology. 17:3-12.

35. Koshihara Y., Neichi T., Murota S., Lao A., Fujimoto Y., Tatsuno T. 1984. Caffeic acid is a selective inhibitor for leukotriene biosynthesis. Biochimica et Biophysica Acta. 792(1):92-7.

36. Turova A. D. 1974. In Medicinal plants of the U. S. S. R. Moscow: Medicine Press Publisher. P72.

37. Motoyashiki T., Miyake M., Morita T., Mizutani K., Masuda H., Ueki H. 1998. Enhancement of the vanadate-stimulated release of lipoprotein lipase activity by astilbin from the leaves of Engelhardtia chrysolepis. Biological & Pharmaceutical Bulletin. 21:5 517-9.

38. Han L. K., Ninomiya H., Taniguchi M., Baba K., Kimura Y., Okuda H. 1998. Norepinephrine-augmenting lipolytic effectors from Astilbe thunbergii rhizomes. Journal of Natural Products. 61:8 1006-11.

39. Durmishidze S. B., Shalashvili A. G., Mjavanadze V. V., Tziklauri G. C. 1981. Flavonoids in several plants of the Georgian republic. P. 194 Tbilisi, Republic of Georgia. Georgia Press.

40. Nardini M., Natella F., Gentili V., Di Felice M., Scaccini C. 1997. Effect of caffeic acid dietary supplementation on the antioxidant defense system in rat: an in vivo study. Archives of Biochemistry and Biophysics. 1; 342(1):157-160.

41. Thiel K. D., Wutzler P., Helbig B., Klocking R., Sprossig M., Schweizer H. 1984. Antiviral effect of enzymatically and nonenzymatically oxidized caffeic and hydrocaffeic acids against Herpesvirus hominis type 1 and type 2 in vitro. Pharmazie. November;39(11):781-2.

42. Kreis W., Kaplan M. H., Freeman J., Sun D. K., Sarin P. S. 1990. Inhibition of HIV replication by Hyssop officinalis extracts. Antiviral Research. December;14(6):323-37.

43. Robinson W. E., Cordeiro M., Abdel-Malek S., Jia Q., Chow S., Reinecke M., Mitchell W. M. 1999. Dicaffeoylquinic acid inhibitors of human immunodeficiency virus integrase: inhibition of the core catalytic domain of human immunodeficiency virus integrase. Molecular Pharmacology. October;50(4): 846-55.

44. Cignarella A., Nastasi M., Cavalli E., Puglisi L. 1996. Novel lipid-lowering properties of Vaccinium myrtillus L. leaves, a traditional antidiabetic treatment, in several models of rat dyslipidaemia: a comparison with ciprofibrate. Thrombosis Research. December1;84(5):311-22.

45. Abidoff M. 1999. Evaluation of glucose lowering properties of blueberry leaves extract. Part 1: Double blind placebo controlled study for the Russian Ministry for National Defense Industries. Part 2. Effect of blueberry leaves extract on plasma glucose level in Type II diabetics. February 1999 - December 1999.

46. Abidoff M. 1999. Identification of major phenolic constituents in blueberry leaves extract (Vaccinium arctostaphylos L) and its effect on human glucose: Double-blind placebo controlled clinical study. Russian Center for Modern Medicine. 1999.

47. Niwa T., Doi U., Kato Y., Osawa T. 1999. Inhibitory mechanism of sinapinic acid against peroxynitrite-mediated tyrosine nitration of protein in vitro. FEBS Letters. October 1;459(1):43-6

48. Kono Y., Shibata H., Kodama Y., Sawa Y. 1995. The suppression of the N-nitrosating reaction by chlorogenic acid. The Biochemical Journal. Devember15;312 (Pt3):947-953.

49. Tsuchiya T., Suzuki O., Igarashi K. 1996. Protective effects of chlorogenic acid on paraquat-induced oxidative stress in rats. Bioscience, Biotechnology, and Biochemistry. 60(5):765-8.

50. Iwahashi H., Negoro Y., Ikeda A., Morishita H., Kido R. 1986. Inhibition by chlorogenic acid of haematin-catalysed retinoic acid 5,6- epoxidation. The Biochemical Journal. November1;239(3):641-6.

51. Shimizu M., Yoshimi N., Yamada Y., Matsunaga K., Kawabata K., Hara A., Moriwaki H., Mori H. 1999. Suppressive effects of chlorogenic acid on N-methyl-N-nitrosourea-induced glandular stomach carcinogenesis in male F344 rats. The Journal of Toxicological Sciences. 24(5):433-9.

52. Mori H., Tanaka T., Shima H., Kuniyasu T., Takahashi M. 1986. Inhibitory effect of chlorogenic acid on methylazoxymethanol acetate-induced carcinogenesis in large intestine and liver of hamsters. Cancer Letters. 30 (1):49-54.

53. Kerry N., and Rice-Ewans C. 1999. Inhibition of peroxynitrite-mediated oxidation of Dopamine by flavonoid and phenolic antioxidants and their structural relationships. The Journal of Neuroscience. July;73(1):247-253.

54. Krasik E., Morozova E., Petrova K. 1970. New results on depression therapy using Rhodiola rosea extract. In Modern Problems of Psychopharmacology. Kemerovo. Pp. 298-300.

55. Krasik E., Petrova K., Ragulina G. 1970. Adaptogenic and stimulative effect of Rhodiola rosea extract. Proceedings of All Union Conference of Neuropathologists and Psychiatrists. Sverdlovsk. May 26-29. Pp. 215-217.

56. Germano C. and Ramazanov Z. 1999. In Arctic Root (Rhodiola Rosea) The Powerful New Ginseng Alternative. New York. Kensington Publishing Corporation.

57. Saratikov A. 1974. Golden Root (Rhodiola rosea). Tomsk. P. 155.

58. Saratikov A., and Krasnov E. A. 1987. Rhodiola rosea is a valuable Medicinal Plant. Tomsk. P.252.

59. Kaliko I. and Tarosova A. 1965. Effect of natural stimulants of the central nervous system. Proceedings of the 3rd Scientific Conference of Physiologists, Biochemists and Pharmacists. Tomsk; Tomsk Medical Sciences University. Pp.302-303.

60. Kaliko I. and Tarasova N. 1966. Effect of extracts of Leuzea and Golden Root on the dynamic characteristics of the central nervous system. Tomsk: Tomsk Medical Sciences University. 1:115-120.

61. Zapuskalova. 1962. Russian Journal of Central Nervous System Function. 1:184-185

62. Ramazanov Z. and Suarez M. 1999. In New Secrets of Effective Natural Stress and Weight Management Using Rhodiola rosea and Rhododendron caucasicum. East Cannan, CT. ATN/Safe Goods Publishing. P. 60-61.

63. Oleynichenko V. F. 1966. Effect of Eleutherococcus and Rhodiola rosea (Golden Root) on hearing of employees of Tomsk electrochemical factory and pilots at Tomsk International Airport. In Natural Stimulators of Central Nervous System. Tomsk. Pp. 124-127

64. Abidoff M. 1997. Stimulative effect of Rhodiola rosea and Rhododendron caucasicum extract on fatty acid release in healthy volunteers. Clinical study for Russian Ministry of Health. Press release of clinical study. Moscow. P. 12.

65. Seifulla. 1999. Sport Pharmacology Manual. Department of Medico-Biological Problems at the Russian Institute for Highest Sports Achievements, National

Research Institute of Physical Culture and Sport of Russian Federation. VNI-IFK - Moscow, Russia.

66. Cherdinzev S. 1971. Doctoral Thesis. Uzbekistan Academy of Sciences. Tashkent, U. S. S. R.

67. Ramazanov Z. and Suarez M. 1999. In New Secrets of Effective Natural Stress and Weight Management Using Rhodiola rosea and Rhododendron caucasicum. East Cannan, CT. ATN/Safe Goods Publishing. P. 56-57.

68. Mandal S., and Stoner G. D. 1990. Inhibition of N-nitrosobenzyl-methylamine-induced esophageal tumorigenesis in rats by ellagic acid. Carcinogenesis. January;11(1):55-61.

69. Chang R. L., Hùang M. T., Wood A.W., Wong C. Q., Newmark H. L., Yagi H., Sayer J. M., Jerina D., Conney A. H. 1985. Effect of ellagic acid and hydroxylated flavonoids on the tumorigenicity of benzo(a)pyrene and (")-78ß,8a-dihydroxy-9a,10a-epoxy-7,8,9,10 tetrahydrobenzo(a) pyrene on mouse skin and in the newborn mouse. Carcinogenesis. August;6(8):1127-1133.

70. Narayanan A., Geoffroy O., Willingham M., Re Gian., Nixon D. 1999. p53/p21 (WAF1/CIP1) expression and its possible role in G1 arrest and apoptosis in ellagic acid treated cancer cells. Cancer Letters. 136:215-221.

71. Narayanan B. A., Re G. G. 2001. IGF-II down regulation associated cell cycle arrest in colon cancer cells exposed to phenolic antioxidant ellagic acid. Anticancer Research. January-February;21(1A):359-64.

72. Narayanan B. A., Narayanan N. K., Stoner G. D., Bullock B. P. 2002. Interactive gene expression pattern in prostate cancer cells exposed to phenolic antioxidants. Life Sciences. March 1;70(15):1821-39.

73. Khanduja K. L., Gandhi R. K., Pathania V., Syal N. 1999. Prevention of N-nitrosodiethylamine-induced lung tumorigenesis by ellagic acid and quercetin in mice. Food and Chemical Toxicology. 37(4):313-8.

74. Constantinou A., Stoner G. D., Mehta R., Rao K., Runyan C., Moon R. 1995. The dietary anticancer agent ellagic acid is a potent inhibitor of DNA topoisomerases in vitro. Nutrition and Cancer. 23(2): 121-30.

75. Aviram, M., Dornfeld, L., Rosenblat M., Volkova N., Kaplan M., Coleman R., Hayek T., Presser D., Fuhrman B. 2000a. Pomegranate juice consumption reduces oxidative stress, atherogenic modifications to LDL, and platelet aggregation: studies in humans and in atherosclerotic apolipoprotein E-deficient mice. American Journal of Clinical Nutrition. May;71(6):1062-76.

76. Shahidi F., Wanasundara P. D., Hong C. 1992. Antioxidant activity of phenolic compounds in meat model system. In Phenolic compounds in food and their effect of health. ACS Symposium, Series 506 Washington, D. C., pp. 214-222.

77. Cai L., and Wu C. D. 1996. Compounds from Syzygium aromaticum possessing growth inhibitory activity against oral pathogens. Journal of Natural Products. 59(10):987-90.

78. GAS (Georgian Academy of Sciences). 2001. Main data base of natural resources. The commission studying productive forces and natural resources at the Presidium of Academy of Sciences of Georgia. http://www.acnet.ge/resources/natresursing.html

79. GIZO. 2002. Georgia. http://www.skategoal.com/gizo_org/gizo.htm

80. EG (Expo Georgia). 2002. About Georgia: Mineral and Energy Resources. http://www.expo.com.ge/georgia.htm

81. Benet S. 1976. In How to live to be 100. The life-style of the people of the Caucasus. P. 100-101. New York. The Dial Press.
82. Boudinot S. 2003. Anatomy of the Gastrointestinal Tract and Drug Absorption. http://chemcases.com/pheno/pheno14.htm
83. Marieb E. N. 1995. In Human anatomy and physiology. Redwood City, California. The Benjamin/Cummings Publishing Company, Inc. Pp. 940-946 .
84. Tortora G. and Anagnostakos N. 1990. In Principles of Anatomy and Physiology. New York: Biological Sciences Textbooks, Inc., A & P Textbooks, Inc., and Elia-Sparta, Inc., Harper Collins Publishers. Pp. 39-42.
85. Draper A. 2001. Case study #5: Disinfection of drinking water. Chem 360, Advanced Environmental Chemistry. http://www.facstaff.bucknell.edu/adraper/360case5.html
86. King W., Dodds L., Allen A. 2000. Relation between stillbirth and specific chlorination by-products in public water supplies. Environmental Health Perspectives. Sep;108(9):883-6.
87. Marieb E. N. 1995. In Human anatomy and physiology. Redwood City, California. The Benjamin/Cummings Publishing Company, Inc. Pp. 813-829.
88. Tortora G. and Anagnostakos N. 1990. In Principles of Anatomy and Physiology. New York: Biological Sciences Textbooks, Inc., A & P Textbooks, Inc., and Elia-Sparta, Inc., Harper Collins Publishers. Pp. 759-775.
89. East Carolina University and Tribbles G. 1999. What are Bacteroides? http://borg.med.ecu.edu/~webpage/about.html
90. Tribbles G. 1999. Development of a Model of Transposition for the Bacteroides Mobilizable Transposon TN4555. Introduction to doctoral thesis. http://borg.med.ecu.edu/~webpage/about.html
91. Mason P. 2001. Probiotics and prebiotics. The Pharmaceutical Journal. 266(7132):118-121.
92. Kimball J. W. 2003. The Human Gastrointestinal (GI) Tract. http://users.rcn.com/jkimball.ma.ultranet/BiologyPages/G/GITract.html
93. Mitsuoka T. 1996. Intestinal flora and human health. Asia Pacific Journal of Clinical Nutrition. 5(1):2-9.
94. Elmer G. 2001. Probiotics: "Living drugs." American Journal of Health-System Pharmacy. June 15;58(12):1101-9.
95. Isolauri E. 2001. Probiotics in human disease. American Journal of Clinical Nutrition. June; 73(6):1142S.
95. Vanderhoof J. 2001. Probiotics: future directions. American Journal of Clinical Nutrition. June;73(6): 1152S.
96. Adderly B. 2002. Life Begets Life. In the News. BluePrint for Health. http://blueprint.bluecrossmn.com/article/bellhowell/101914938
97. Vanderhoof J. and Young R. J. 2002. Bacterial overgrowth. The Oley Foundation. University of Nebraska Medical Center, Creighton University. http://www.c4isr.com/oley/lifeline/bacter.html
98. Bongaerts G. and Severijnen R. 2001. The beneficial, antimicrobial effect of probiotics. Medical Hypotheses. 56(2):174-177.
99. Gill H., Cross M., Rutherfurd K., Gopal P. 2001. Dietary probiotic supplementation to enhance cellular immunity in the elderly. British Journal of Biomedical Science. 58(2):94-6
100. Rolfe R. D. 2000. The role of probiotic cultures in the control of gastrointestinal health. Journal of Nutrition. 130:396S-402S.

101. Borody T. J. 2000. "Flora Power" – fecal bacteria cure chronic C. difficile diarrhea. The American Journal of Gastroenterology. November;95(11):3028-9.
102. Catto-Smith A. G. 1996. Gut flora and mucosal function. Asia Pacific Journal of Clinical Nutrition. 5(1):36-38.
103. Andrews P. J., Barnes P., Borody T. J. 1992. Chronic constipation reversed by restoration of bowel flora. A case and a hypothesis. European Journal of Gastroenterology and Hepatology. 4:245-7.
104. Andrews P. J. and Borody T. J. 1993. Putting back the bugs: Bacterial treatment relieves chronic constipation and symptoms of irritable bowel syndrome. Medical Journal of Australia. 159:633-4.
105. Majamaa H. and Isolauri E. 1997. Probiotics: a novel approach in the management of food allergy. The Journal of Allergy and Clinical Immunology. February;99(2):179-185.
106. Stedman T. L. 1995. In Stedman's Medical Dictionary. Baltimore. Williams & Wilkins. 26th edition. P. 1312.
107. Marieb E. N. 1995. In Human anatomy and physiology. Redwood City, California. The Benjamin/Cummings Publishing Company, Inc. P. G-13.
108. Arora, G. 2003. Telephone interview of Gulshan Arora, Ph.D., by the author, Shaffer Fox. May 2.
109. Kneifel W. and Mayer H. 1991. Vitamin profiles of kefirs made from milks of different species. International Journal of Food Sciences and Technology. 26:423-428.
110. Anfiteatro D. M. 2003. A Probiotic Gem Cultured with a Probiotic Jewel...Kefir Grains! Mountains and Flowers of North Caucasus. Dom's Kefir In-Site. April 29. http://users.chariot.net.au/~dna/kefirpage.html
111. Fox W. S. and Ramazanov Z. 1997. Rhododendron caucasicum product information brochure: Total Health for the Total Body.
112. PM. (PubMed). 2002. Keyword searches: exercise; diet. National Center for Biotechnology Information, National Library of Medicine, National Institutes of Health. http://www.ncbi.nlm.nih.gov/entrez/query
113. Rohack J. J. 1997. Report of the council on medical education: nutritional and dietetic education for medical students. AMA-CME Report March 1. http://www.ama-asn.org/meetings/public/int97/cmer03.htm
114. Anding J. 2000. Nutri-facts. Texas Agricultural Extension Service; The Texas A & M University System. January; Issue 3.
115. NHLBI (National Hearth, Lung, and Blood Institute). 2001. How you can lower your cholesterol. National Institutes of Health. http://www.nhlbi.nih.gov/chd/Tipsheets/vfitness.htm
116. McClam E. 2002. Feds Say 70 Percent Not Exercising. Associated Press. http://www.washingtonpost.com/wp-dyn/articles/A8953-2002Aprl7.html
117. CDC (Centers for Disease Control and Prevention). 2002a. Leisure-time physical activity among adults: United States, 1997-98. Advance Data. 325: April 7.
118. Ramazanov Z. and Suarez M. 1999. In New Secrets of Effective Natural Stress and Weight Management Using Rhodiola rosea and Rhododendron caucasicum. . East Cannan, CT. ATN/Safe Goods Publishing. P. 29-31.

CHAPTER 3. RHODODENDRON CAUCASICUM

1. Ramazanov Z. and Suarez M. 1999. In New Secrets of Effective Natural Stress and Weight Management Using Rhodiola rosea and Rhododendron caucasicum. East Cannan, CT. ATN/Safe Goods Publishing. P. 14,15.
2. Ramazanov Z. 2000. Data provided to the author, Shaffer Fox.
3. CIE (Compton's Interactive Encyclopedia). 1999. Rhododendron.
4. RSF. (Rhododendron Species Foundation.) 2002. Rhododendron Species. http://www.rhodygarden.org/2RHSPE.html
5. Durmishidze S. V., Shalashvilee A. G., Mzhavanadze V. V., Tsiklauree G. C. 1981. In Flavonoids and Oxycinnamic Acids in Some Species of Georgia Wild Flora. Tblisi. Metsniereba. Chapter 1. Flavonoids in Rhododendron Caucasian and Rhododendron Pontific.
6. Kemertelidze E. 2003. History of the Institute of Pharmacochemistry of the Georgian Academy of Sciences.
7. Rossiisskiy D. M. 1954. Rhododendron as a cardiovascular remedy. Pharmacology and Toxicology. Volume 4.
8. Ramazanov Z. 1997, 2000, 2001, 2002, 2003, 2004. Telephone interviews of Zakir Ramazanov, Ph.D., by the author, Shaffer Fox.
9. Abidoff M. 1997. Rhododendron caucasicum: pharmacology and phytochemistry. Moscow. Center for Modern Medicine.
10. Hagerman A. E. 2002. Tannin Chemistry. http://www.users.muohio.edu/hagermanae/tannin.pdf
11. Turova A. D., Pogorelova A., Ovchinikkova A., Golovleva A. 1950. Rhododenzid: a new heart disease drug from rhododendron. Pharmacology and Toxicology. 13:31-37.
12. Rossiisskiy D. M. 1954. Clinical study of in-hospital treatment of cardio-vascular insufficiency by Rhododendron preparations. (Two clinical studies conducted for the U. S. S. R. Health Department.)
13. Rossiisskiy D. M. 1954. Rhododendron: a new remedy for regulation of blood circulation deficiency. Pharmacology and Toxicology. 17:3-12.
14. Gedevanishvili D. M., and Tzereteli M. P. 1955. Specific physiological effect of Rhododendron. Proceedings of Georgian Pharmaceutical Institute. 2:22.
15. Gvishiani G. C. 1955. Rhodogern – extract of Rhododendron in treatments of high blood pressure. International Congress on pathology of cardio-vascular systems. Pavlov Institute of Physiology, Leningrad, U. S. S. R.
16. Bostanashvili B. S., and Kemertelidze E. P. 1956. Effect of Rhododendron caucasicum Ungern extract on the regulation of blood pressure. Proceedings of Pharmaceutical Institute of the Georgian Academy of Sciences. 8:25-26.
17. Gedevanishvili D. M., and Tzereteli M. P. 1956. Pharmacology of Rhododendron. Proceedings of Georgian Pharmaceutical Institute. Pp. 85-90.
18. Gedevanishvili D. M., and Tzereteli M. P. 1960. Pharmacological effect of glycosides of Rhododendron. Proceedings of Georgian Pharmaceutical Institute. Pp. 17-27.
19. Smith M. L. 2002. Definition provided by Marjorie Smith, M. D., during a telephone interview by the author, Shaffer Fox. November 18.
20. Fox W. S. 1997. Rhododendron caucasicum information audio tape. An interview of Dr. Zakir Ramazanov. Russia's 2000 Year Old Secret Revealed.

21. N. F. (Nobel Foundation). 2004. Albert Szent-Gyorgyi – Biography. http://www.nobel.se/medicine/laureates/1937/szent-gyorgyi-bio.htm/
22. M. B. L. (Marine Biological Laboratory). 2001. Albert Szent-Gyorgyi (1893-1986). http://www.hpo.hu/English/inventor/eszgyalb.html
23. Szent-Gyorgyi A. 1937. Oxidation, energy transfer, and vitamins. Nobel Lecture. December 11. http://www.nobel.se/medicine/laureates/ 1937/szent-gyorgyi-lecture.pdf
24. Goldstein J. L. 1996. Albert Lasker Award for Basic Medical Research, 1996. Comments at the Awards Ceremony. http://www.laskerfoundation.org/awards/library/1996b_pp.shtml
25. Passwater R. A. 2002. Bioflavonoids, "Vitamin P" and Inflammation: An interview with Dr. Miklos Gabor. Whole Foods Magazine.
26. Smith T. J. 1999. In Renewal: The Anti-Aging Revolution. New York. St. Martins Paperbacks. P. 315-338
27. Durmishidze S. V. and Nutzubidze N. N. 1954. Method of the investigation of tannins using chromatography. Proceedings of the Soviet Academy of Sciences. 96: 1197.
28. Kemertelidze E. P. 2003. Telephone interview of E. P. Kemertelidze, D. Sc., by the author, Shaffer Fox. July 24.
29. Shalashvili A. 1967. Method of total flavonoids extraction from Rhododendron caucasicum. Proceedings of the Georgian Academy of Sciences. 48:603.
30. Shalashvili A. 1967. Flavonoids of Rhododendron caucasicum. Proceedings of the Georgian Academy of Sciences. 46:115.
31. Shalashvili A. 1973. Identification of flavonoids in Rhododendron caucasicum. Plant Biochemistry. 1:214.
32. Thieme H., Walewska E., Winkler H. J. 1969. Isolation of salidroside from leaves of Rhododendron ponticum x catawbiense. Pharmazie. December 12; 24(12):783.
33. Ye Y. C., Chen Q. M., Jin K. P., hou S. X., Chai F. L. Hai P. 1993. Effect of salidroside on cultured myocardial cells anoxia/reoxygenation injuries. Hongguo Yao Li Xue Bao. September;14(5):424-6.
34. Brown R. P., Gerbarg P. L., Ramazanov Z. 2002. Rhodiola rosea: A Phytomedicinal Overview. HerbalGram 56. http://herbalgram.org
35. Abidoff M. & Kekelidze N. 1997. Effect of Rhododendron caucasicum herbal supplement on dietary fat absorption and weight loss in obese patients. Moscow Center for Modern Medicine. February 12.
36. Brown W. 2002. In the Beginning: Compelling Evidence for Creation and the Flood. Life Sciences. Center for Scientific Creation. http://www.creation-science.com/onlinebook/PartI3.html
37. Roper G. C. 1997. Molecule. The Grolier Multimedia Encyclopedia. Grolier Interactive, Inc.
38. Feinberg G. 1997. Atom. The Grolier Multimedia Encyclopedia. Grolier Interactive, Inc.
39. Feinberg G. 1997. Electron. The Grolier Multimedia Encyclopedia. Grolier Interactive, Inc.
40. Cooper K. 1994. In Antioxidant Revolution. Nashville. Thomas Nelson, Inc. P.19.
41. McBride J., Porter N., Rüchardt., Smith P., MacKay C. 2000. Moses gomberg in Ann Arbor. http://www.chem.yale.edu/~chem125/125/history99/5Valence/GombergWe b/gomberghouses.htm

42. Wardman P. 1993. Free radicals: nature's way of saying no or molecular murder. Review article from the Gray Laboratory Annual Report, Gray Laboratory Cancer Research Trust.

43. Buettner G. R. and Schafer F. Q. 2000. Free radicals, oxidants, and antioxidants. Teratology. 62:234.

44. Beckman K. B. and Ames B. N. 1998. The free radical theory of aging matures. Physiological Reviews. April;78(2):547-581.

45. Tortora G. and Anagnostakos N. 1990. In Principles of Anatomy and Physiology. New York: Biological Sciences Textbooks, Inc., A & P Textbooks, Inc., and Elia-Sparta, Inc., Harper Collins Publishers. P. 582.

46. Prior R. L., and Cao G. 1999. Variability in dietary antioxidant related natural product supplements: the need for method of standardization. JANA Vol. 2. Pp. 46-56.

47. Teselkin I. O., Zhambalova B. A., Babenkova I. V., Tiukavkina N. A. 1996. Antioxidant properties of dihydroquercetin. Biofizika. 41(3):620-4.

48. Tiukavkina N. A., Rulenko I. A., Kolesnik I. A. 1996. Natural flavonoids as dietary antioxidants and biologically active additives. (Moscow) Nutrition. (2):33-8.

49. AOA (American Obesity Association). 2002. Obesity in the U. S. http://www.obesity.org/subs/fastfacts/obesity_US.shtml

50. CDC (Centers for Disease Control and Prevention). 2002e. Section III, Risk factors and use of preventive services, United States: Overweight among adults. http://www.cdc.gov/nccdphp/burdenbook2002/03_overadult.htm

51. NIDDK. (The National Institute of Diabetes and Digestive and Kidney Diseases). 2000. Statistics related to overweight and obesity. The National Institutes of Health. http://www.niddk.nih.gov/health/nutrit/pubs/statobes.htm

52. Flegal K. M., Carroll M. D., Kuczmarski R. J., Johnson C. L. 1998. Overweight and obesity in the United States: prevalence and trends, 1960-1994. International Journal of Obesity and Related Metabolic Disorders. January;22(1):39-47.

53. Mokdad A. H., Serdula M. K., Dietz W. H., Bowman B. A., Marks J. S., Koplan J. P. 2001. The spread of the obesity epidemic in the United States, 1991-1998. Journal of the American Medical Association. June 20;285(23):2973.

54. NIDDK and NHLBI (National Institute of Diabetes and Digestive and Kidney Diseases, and the National Heart, Lung, and Blood Institute). 1998. Executive summary: Clinical guidelines on the identification, evaluation, and treatment of overweight and obesity in adults: Obesity Education Initiative National Task Force on Prevention and Treatment of Obesity; North American Association for the Study of Obesity. American Journal of Clinical Nutrition. 68:899-917.

55. Satcher D. 1998. Childhood Obesity: Causes & Prevention. Opening remarks. October 27. http://www.usda.gov/cnpp/Seminars/obesity.PDF

56. Anand, R. 1998. Childhood Obesity: Causes & Prevention. Symposium Proceedings. Forward. October 27. http://www.usda.gov/cnpp/Seminars/obesity.PDF

57. Reuters. 2003. Even U. S. Toddlers Are Obese. Washington, D. C. Reuters. May 5.

58. Mendler M. and Schoenfield L. J. 2004. Fatty Liver: Nonalcoholic Fatty Liver Disease (NAFLD) and Nonalcoholic Steatohepatitis (NASH). http://www.medicinenet.com/Fatty_Liver/page1.htm

59. Sinha R., Fisch G., Teague B., Tamborlane W. V., Banyas B., Allen K., Savo M.,

Rieger V., Taksali S., Barbetta G., Sherwin R. S., Caprio S. 2002. Prevalence of impaired glucose tolerance among children and adolescents with marked obesity. New England Journal of Medicine. March14;346(11):854-5.

60. BBC. (BBC News). 2002. Diabetes threat to children. February 21. http://news.bbc.co.uk/hi/english/health/newsid_1827000/1827822.stm

61. BBC. (BBC News). 2002. Obese children heading for diabetes. March 14. http://news.bbc.co.uk/hi/english/health/newsid_1871000/1871532.stm

62. BBC. (BBC News). 2002. Syndrome X the 'silent killer. April 16. http://news.bbc.co.uk/hi/english/health/newsid_1933000/1933706.stm

63. Michaud D. S., Liu S., Giovannucci E., Willett W. C., Colditz G. A., Fuchs C. S. 2002. Dietary sugar, glycemic load, and pancreatic cancer risk in a prospective study. Journal of the National Cancer Institute. September 4;94(17):1293-300.

64. Challem J. 2000. Syndrom X. http://www.syndrome-x.com

65. Simao P. 2002. CDC: More adults reporting high blood pressure. Reuters. June 8

66. CDC (Centers for Disease Control and Prevention). 2002. Obesity and overweight, Obesity trends: Prevalence among U. S. adults of a metabolic syndrom associated with obesity. Findings from the third NHANES III survey. http://www.cdc.gov/nccdphp/dnpa/obesity/trend/metabolic.htm

67. AACE (American Association of Clinical Endocrinologists). 2002. Findings and recommendations from the American College of Endocrinology Conference on the Insulin Resistance Syndrome. http://www.aace.com/pub/BMI/findings.php

68. Fox M. 2002. Insulin syndrome affects a third of U. S. – report. Reuters. August 27.

69. BBC (BBC News). 2002. Starchy diet 'linked to cancer.' September 4. http://news.bbc.co.uk/2/hi/health/2236473.stm

70. Calle E. E., Rodriguez C., Walker-Thurmond K., Thun M. J. 2003. Overweight, obesity, and mortality from cancer in a prospectively studied cohort of U. S. adults. The New England Journal of Medicine. April 24. 348(17):1625-38.

71. McConnaughey J. 2003. Losing Weight May Prevent Cancer Deaths. Washington, D. C. The Associated Press. April 23.

72. Tanner L. 2003. Study: Obesity Ups Risk of Birth Defects. Washington, D. C. The Associated Press. May 5.

73. Watkins M. L., Rasmussen S. A., Honein M. A., Botto L. D., Moore C. A. 2003. Maternal obesity and risk for birth defects. . Pediatrics. May. 111(5 Part 2):1152-8.

74. CDC (Centers for Disease Control and Prevention). 2002. Section III, Risk factors and use of preventive services, United States: Overweight among adults. http://www.cdc.gov/nccdphp/burdenbook2002/03_overadult.htm

75. Allison D. B., Sanders S. E. 2000. Obesity in North America. An overview. Medical Clinics of North America. March;84(2):305-32.

76. Anand, R. 1998. Childhood Obesity: Causes & Prevention. Symposium Proceedings. Forward. October 27. http://www.usda.gov/cnpp/Seminars/obesity.PDF

77. Fox M. 2002. Supersize portions fattening U. S. Reuters. June 18.

78. Chapus C., Rovery M., Sarda L., Verger R. 1988. Minireview of pancreatic lipase and colipase. Biochimie. 70:1223-34.

79. Carey M. C., and Hernell O. 1992. Digestion and absorption of fat. Seminars in Gastrointestinal Disease. 3:189-208.

80. Hernell O. 1999. Assessing fat absorption. Journal of Pediatrics. 135:4:407-9.
81. DeCaro A., Figarella C., Amic J., Michel R., Guy O. 1977. Human pancreatic lipase: a glycoprotein. Biochimica et Biophysica Acta. 490:411-19.
82. Kalivianakis M. 2002. Dietary lipids. http://www.ub.rug.nl/eldoc/dis/medicine/m.kalivianakis/c1.pdf
83. Reagan J. 2002. Stamina – Nutrition Connection. In Executive Wellness: A Guide for Senior Leaders. Carlisle Barracks, PA. U. S. Army Physical Fitness Research Institute. U. S. Army War College. http://www.hooah4health.com/body/staminanutrition.htm
84. McBride J. 2001. Low-fat foods can help lower fat intake. Agricultural Research Service. U. S. D. A. October 1. http://www.ars.usda.gov/is/pr/2001/011001.htm
85. Ramazanov Z. and Suarez M. 1999. In New Secrets of Effective Natural Stress and Weight Management Using Rhodiola rosea and Rhododendron caucasicum. East Cannan, CT. ATN/Safe Goods Publishing. P. 26-28
86. Haller C. and Benowitz N. 2000. Adverse cardiovascular and central nervous system events associated with dietary supplements containing ephedra alkaloids. New England Journal of Medicine. Dec 21;343(25):1886-7.
87. MDN (MDNews). 2000. Ephedra use associated with serious health risks. http://praxis.md/newsbureau/MD/newsarchive.asp?news_id=2595&news=MD
88. McKinney M. 2000. Even modest weight loss reduces diabetes risk. New York. Reuters Health Information. May 04.
89. Zazinski J. 2000. Small loss is a big gain. Boston University Research Briefs.
90. Motoyashiki T., Miyake M., Morita T., Mizutani K., Masuda H., Ueki H. 1998. Enhancement of the vanadate stimulated release of lipoprotein lipase activity by astilbin from the leaves of Engelhardtia chrysolepis. Biological & Pharmaceutical Bulletin. 21:5 517-9.
91. Han L. K., Ninomiya H., Taniguchi M., Baba K., Kimura Y., Okuda H. 1998. Norepinephrine-augmenting lipolytic effectors from Astilbe thunbergii rhizomes. Journal of Natural Products. 61:8 1006-11.
92. Tortora G. and Anagnostakos N. 1990. In Principles of Anatomy and Physiology. New York: Biological Sciences Textbooks, Inc., A & P Textbooks, Inc., and Elia-Sparta, Inc., Harper Collins Publishers. P. 573.
93. Burns G. 1997. Heart, animal. The Grolier Multimedia Encyclopedia. Grolier Interactive, Inc.
94. Frazier O. 1997. Heart, human. The Grolier Multimedia Encyclopedia. Grolier Interactive, Inc.
95. U of M (University of Michigan). 2001. Disease Management: Heart Valve Diseases. http://www.med.umich.edu/cvc/adult/dishea.htm
96. Marieb E. N. 1995. In Human Anatomy and Physiology. Redwood City, California. The Benjamin/Cummings Publishing Company, Inc. P. 619-622.
97. DeRoin D. A. 2004. Information About Common Heart Diseases: Heart Murmur. http://www.temple.edu/heart/html/murmur.html
98. BHC and HRC (Better Health Channel and Heart Research Center). 2003. Heart Murmur.
99. CCM (Cardiovascular Consultants of Maine, P .A.). What is Mitral Valve Prolapse? http://www.heartmaine.com
100. TMM (The Merck Manual). Mitral Valve Disease. http://www.merck.com/mrk-shared/mmanual/section16/chapter207/207b.jsp

101. SD (Surgery Door). Mitral Valve Disease: What is Mitral Valve Disease? www. surgerydoor.co.uk/medical_conditions/Indices/M/mitral_valve_disease.htm
102. UHLNHST (University Hospitals of Leicester NHS trust). 2002. Mitral Valve Disease. http://www.yourheart.org.uk/mitral.php
103. WH (Wockhardt Hospital). 2004. Valve Disease. http://www.whhi.com/valve.html
104. PDR (PDR Family Guide to Women's Health and Prescription Drugs). 2003. Heart Disease: The Greatest Threat of All. http://www.pdrhealth.com/content/women_health/chapters/fgwh12.shtml
105. Marieb E. N. 1995. In Human Anatomy and Physiology. Redwood City, California. The Benjamin/Cummings Publishing Company, Inc. P. 639,640.
106. MCP (Mercy Health Partners). 2003. Mitral Valve Disease: General Overview. http://www.mercyweb.org/heartcenter/html/hvd_detail.asp?ContentId=114
107. AHA (American Heart Association). 2001. Mitral Valve and Mitral Valve Prolapse. http://www.americanheart.org/Heart_and _Stroke_A_Z_Guide/mitral.html
108. AHA (American Heart Association). 2002. Mitral Valve and Mitral Valve Prolapse. http://www.americanheart.org/presenter.jhtml?identifier=4717
109. MVPCA (The Mitral Valve Prolapse Center of Alabama). 2001. What are the symptoms of MVP? MVP Symptoms and Testing. 7/27/10. http://www.mvprolapse.com/symtest.htm
110. SMVPS (The Society for MVP Syndrome). 2001. Help is available for mitral valve prolapse syndrome! http://www.mitralvalveprolapse.com
111. HIN (Heart Information Network). 1997. Mitral valve prolapse: The most common heart valve abnormality. http://www.heartinfo.com/news97/mvp82697.htm
112. Ramazanov Z. and Suarez M. 1999. In New Secrets of Effective Natural Stress and Weight Management Using Rhodiola rosea and Rhododendron caucasicum. East Cannan, CT. ATN/Safe Goods Publishing. P. 46,47.
113. Abu-Amsha R., Croft K. D., Puddley I. B., Proudfoot J. M. Beilin L. 1996. Phenolic content of various beverages determines the extent of inhibition of human serum and low-density lipoprotein oxidation in vitro: identification and mechanism of action of some cinnamic acid derivatives from red wine. Clinical Science (London). October;91(4):449-58.
114. Vieira O., Escargueil-Blanc I., Meilhac O., Basile J. P., Laranjinha J., Almeida L., Salvayre R., Negre-Salvayre A. 1998. Effect of dietary phenolic compounds on apoptosis of human cultured endothelial cells induced by oxidized LDL. British Journal of Pharmacology; 123(3):565-573.
115. Kim Dong-Wook, Bang Kyu-Ho, Roh Sung-Bae, Park Won-Hwan, Kim Cheorl-Ho. 2001. Inhibitory effect of chlorogenic acid on LDL oxidation and foam cell formation. Poster Session. The Biochemical Society of the Republic of Korea. October 18.
116. Nardini M., D'Aquino M., Tomassi G., Gentili V., Di Felice M., Scaccini C. 1995. Inhibition of human low-density lipoprotein oxidation by caffeic acid and other hydroxycinnamic acid derivatives. Free Radical Biology & Medicine. 19(5):541-52.
117. Guthrie P. 2002. Study: One in three adults suffers from arthritis. Arthritis Foundation. Cox News Service. The Atlanta Journal Constitution. October 25. http://www.arthritis.org/Resources/DisplayScreamingNews.asp?id=269

118. CDC (Centers for Disease Control and Prevention). 2001b. Arthritis: The nation's leading cause of disability. http://www.scs.gov/nccdphp/arthritis/index.htm
119. AF (Arthritis Foundation). 2001. Osteoarthritis (OA). www.arthritis.org/answers/DiseaseCenter/oa.asp
120. CHR (Calgary Health Region). 2000. Your Health: Osteoarthritis. http://www.crha-health.ab.ca/hlthconn/items/osteoart.htm
121. Marieb E. N. 1995. In Human anatomy and physiology. Redwood City, California. The Benjamin/Cummings Publishing Company, Inc. P. 241-245.
122. AAOS (American Academy of Orthopedic Surgeons). 2000. Arthritis. http://orthoinfo.aaos.org/brochure/thr_report.cfm?Thread_ID=2&topcategory=Arthritis
123. AF (Arthritis Foundation). 2002. Disease center. http://www.arthritis.org/conditions/DiseaseCenter/oa.asp
124. Ramazanov Z. and Suarez M. 1999. In New Secrets of Effective Natural Stress and Weight Management Using Rhodiola rosea and Rhododendron caucasicum. East Cannan, CT. ATN/Safe Goods Publishing. P. 48-50.
125. Ramazanov Z. 1997. Data provided to the author, Shaffer Fox
126. NIAMS (National Institute of Arthritis and Musculoskeletal and Skin Diseases. 2002. Questions and Answers About Gout. http://www.niams.nih.gov/hi/topics/gout/gout.htm
127. AAA (All About Arthritis). 2000. Gout arthritis: Symptoms, causes and treatments for uric acid buildup. http://www.allaboutarthritis.com/arthritis.cfm/about/164
128. ACR (American College of Rheumatology). 2000. Gout. http://www.rheumatology.org/patients/factsheet/gout.html
129. Ramazanov Z. and Suarez M. 1999i. In New Secrets of Effective Natural Stress and Weight Management Using Rhodiola rosea and Rhododendron caucasicum. East Cannan, CT. ATN/Safe Goods Publishing. P. 50-51.
130. Pal B. and Andersen F. 2002. Gout (podagra or uric acid). Netdoctorco.uk. http://www.netdoctor.co.uk/diseases/facts/gout.htm
131. Brewer E. and Cochran K. 1998. What is gout? http://webmd.lycos.com/content/article/4/1680_51325
132. Fox W. S. and Ramazanov Z. 1997. Rhododendron caucasicum information brochure: Total Health for the Total Body.
133. Samartzev A. D., Aushev I. V., Israelov R. R. 1965. Effect of Rhododendron caucasicum extract on gout and sodium release in urine. Dagestan State Hospital Annual Report. P. 112.
134. CIE (Compton's Interactive Encyclopedia). 1999. Minkowski, Oskar.
135. UCDHS (University of California Davis Health System). 2000. What is gout? http://wellness.ucdavis.edu/medical_conditions_az/gout93.html
136. Closa D., Torres M., Hotter G., Bioque G., León OS., Gelpí E., Rósello-Catafau J. 1997. Prostanoids and free radicals in Cl4C-induced hepatotoxicity in rats: effect of astilbin. Prostaglandins, Leukotrienes, and Essential Fatty Acids. 56(4):331-334.
137. Igarashi K., Uchida Y., Murakami N., Mizutani K., Masuda H. 1996. Effect of astilbin in tea processed from leaves of Engelhardtia chrysolepis on the serum and liver lipid concentrations and on the erythrocyte and liver antioxidative enzyme activities of rats. Bioscience, Biotechnology, and Biochemistry. 60(3): 513-5.

138. Marieb E. N. 1995. In Human anatomy and physiology. Redwood City, California. The Benjamin/Cummings Publishing Company, Inc. P. 514.
139. Quigley, H. 1996. Number of people with glaucoma worldwide. British Journal of Ophthalmology. 80(5):389-93.
140. NEI (National Eye Institute). 2001. Healthy vision 2001 – glaucoma. National Institutes of Health, Department of Health and Human Services. 7/25.
141. PBA (Prevent Blindness America). 2001. Glaucoma alert: Waiting for symptoms can lead to vision loss. Prevent Blindness America News. 8 January. http://www.preventblindness.org/news/releases/glaucoma_html
142. TGF (The Glaucoma Foundation). 2002. About glaucoma. http://www.glaucomafoundation.org/education_content.php?i=7
143. Tortora G. and Anagnostakos N. 1990f. In Principles of Anatomy and Physiology. New York: Biological Sciences Textbooks, Inc., A & P Textbooks, Inc., and Elia-Sparta, Inc., Harper Collins Publishers. Pp. 474,490.
144. Wolverton, G. M. 2003. Complications of Diabetes Mellitus. http://www.wolvertonmd.com/diabetescomp.html
145. Riihimaa, Päivi Tossavainen née. 2002. Markers of Microvascular Complications in Adolescents with Type 1 Diabetes. 2.3 Hyperglycaemia in the pathogenesis of microvascular complications. http://herkules.oulu.fi/isbn951426892X/htmlx333.html
146. Musser, J. C. 1997. Chewing Gum. The Grolier Multimedia Encyclopedia. Grolier Interactive, Inc.
147. Fonseca V., Munshi, M., Merin L. M., Bradford J. D. 1996. Diabetic Retinopathy: A Review for the Primary Care Physician. http://www.sma.org/smj/96sept1.htm
148. Haraguchi H., Ohmi I., Fukuda A., Tamura Y., Mizutani K., Tanaka O., Chou W. H. 1997. Inhibition of aldose reductase and sorbitol accumulation by astilbin and taxifolin dihydroflavonols in Engelhardtia chrysolepis. Bioscience, Biotechnology, and Biochemistry. (4):651-4.
149. Haraguchi H., Mochida Y., Sakai S., Masuda H., Tamura Y., Mizutani K., Tanaka O., Chou W. H. 1996. Protection against oxidative damage by dihydroflavonols in Engelhardtia chrysolepis. Bioscience, Biotechnology, and Biochemistry. 60(6): 945-948.
150. Haraguchi H., Ohmi I., Masuda H., Tamura Y., Mizutani K., Tanaka O., Chou W. H. 1996. Inhibition of aldose reductase by dihydroflavonols in Engelhardtia chrysolepis and effects on other enzymes. Experientia. 52(6):564-7.
151. Crockett, L. J. 1997. Bacteria.. The Grolier Multimedia Encyclopedia. Grolier Interactive, Inc.
152. Grundy, W. E. 1999. Bacteria. The Compton Interactive Encyclopedia. The Learning Company, Inc.
153. Fettner A. G. 1997. Bubonic Plague. The Grolier Multimedia Encyclopedia. Grolier Interactive, Inc.
154. Rubin R. J., Harrington C. A., Poon A., Dietrich K., Greene J. A., Moiduddin A. 1999. The economic impact of staphylococcus aureus infection in New York City hospitals. Emerging Infectious Diseases. 5 (1):1-12.
155. CDC (Centers for Disease Control and Prevention). 2003. Disease Information: Group A Streptococcal (GAS) Disease. http://www.dcd.gov/ncidod/dbmd/diseaseinfo/groupastreptococcal_g.htm

156. OHSU Health (Oregon Health & Science University). 2003. Escherichia coli 0157:H7

157. CDC (Centers for Disease Control and Prevention). 1999. Emerging Infectious Diseases. Hospitals Stays Can Be Harmful for Your Health. http://www.cdc.gov/ncidod/eid/press_r/rubin.htm

158. Fisher, I. 1998. Hospitals forge and alliance to fight antibiotic-resistant bacteria. New York Times. June 28.

159. Berens M. J. 2002. Tribune investigation: unhealthy hospitals. Chicago Tribune. July 21. P. 1.

160. Bonner J., and Dunnett B. 1998. Scientists track spread of antibiotic-resistant bacteria in 12 New York City hospitals. Grant from Bristol-Myers Squibb Foundation funds study showing efficacy of a molecular surveillance network. News from The Rockefeller University. July 15.

161. Rubin R. J., Harrington C. A., Poon A., Dietrich K., Greene J. A., Moiduddin A. 1999. The economic impact of staphylococcus aureus infection in New York City hospitals. Emerging Infectious Diseases. 5 (1):1-12.

162. Askari E. 2002. Germs develop a deadly defense: Drug-resistant bacteria discovered in Detroit. Detroit Free Press. http://www.freep.com/news/health/nstaph12_220021112.htm

163. Warner, J. 2003. Bacteria Bigger Threat Than SARS. New York. WebMD Medical News. April 30.

164. Landrault N., Poucheret P., Ravel P., Gase F., Cros G., Teissedre P-L. 2001. Antioxidant capacities and phenolic levels of French wines from different varieties and vintages. Journal of Agricultural and Food Chemistry. 49:3341-3348.

165. Pellegrini N., Simonetti P., Gardana C., Brenna O., Brighenti F., Pietta P. 2000. Polyphenol content and total antioxidant activity of vini novelli (Young Red Wines). Journal of Agricultural and Food Chemistry. 48:732-735.

166. Ramazanov Z. and Suarez M. 1999. In New Secrets of Effective Natural Stress and Weight Management Using Rhodiola rosea and Rhododendron caucasicum. East Cannan, CT. ATN/Safe Goods Publishing. P. 17-20.

167. Woodward A., and Reed J. D. 1997. Nitrogen metabolism of sheep and goats consuming Acacia brevispica and Sesbania sesban. Journal of Animal Science. 75:1130-1139.

168. Zaprametov M. N. 1994. Biochemistry of catechins, biosysnthesis, metabolism and their practical application. Moscow. Science Publisher Press. P. 300.

169. Sterling M. 2000. Proanthocyanidin Power. Nutrition Science News. June.

170. ATSDR (Agency for Toxic Substances and Disease Registry). 1997. Public health statement for chloroform. http://www.atsdr.cdc.gov/toxprofiles/phs6.html

171. ARI (Applied Research Institute). 1998. n-Butanol. Material safety data sheet. http://www.arpltd.com/n-butano.htm

172. KSU (Kansas State University). 2002 Good laboratory safety practices. http://www.ksu.edu/safety/progrm10.htm

CHAPTER 4. CAUCASIAN BLUEBERRY LEAVES

1. Abidoff M. 1999. Identification of major phenolic constituents in blueberry leaves extract (Vaccinium arctostaphylos L) and its effect on human glucose: Double-blind placebo controlled clinical study. Russian Center for Modern Medicine. Internal documents provided to the author, Shaffer Fox.
2. Abidoff M. 1999. Evaluation of glucose lowering properties of blueberry leaves extract. Part 1: Double blind placebo controlled study for the Russian Ministry for National Defense Industries. Part 2. Effect of blueberry leaves extract on plasma glucose level in Type II diabetics. February- December. Internal Documents provided to the author, Shaffer Fox.
3. Ramazanov Z. 2000, 2001, 2002, 2003. Telephone interviews of Zakir Ramazanov, Ph.D., by the author, Shaffer Fox.
4. Mshavanadze V. V. 1971. Chlorogenic acid in Caucasian blueberry leaves (Vaccinium arctostaphylos L). Bulletin of the Georgian Academy of Sciences. 62:189-192.
5. Durmishidze S. B., Shalashvili A. G., Mshavanadze V. V., Tziklauri G. C. 1981. Flavonoids in several plants of the Georgian republic. P. 194 Tbilisi, Republic of Georgia. Georgia Press.
6. del Rio, M. J. 2000. Blueberry Leaves Extract: For Treatment of Diabetes and Prevention of Neurodegenerative Diseases. Position paper forwarded to the author, Shaffer Fox.
7. PM (PubMed). 2002. Keyword searches: caffeic acid, chlorogenic acid, hydroxycinnamic acid. National Center for Biotechnology Information, National Library of Medicine, National Institutes of Health. http://www.ncbi.nlm.nih.gov/entrez/query
8. Mshavanadze V. V., Targamadse I. L., Dranik L. I. 1972. Phenolic compounds in leaves of Vaccinium arctostaphylos L. Chemistry of Natural Products. 1(144): 124.
9. Fox W. S. 2003. Based on the results of five certificates of analysis acquired by the author, Shaffer Fox, between 2001 and 2003.
10. Ramazanov Z. 2000. Data provided to the author, Shaffer Fox.
11. ADA (American Diabetes Association.). 2001. The Dangerous Toll of Diabetes. http://www.diabetes.org/ada/facts.asp
12. CDC (Centers for Disease Control and Prevention). 2001. Twin epidemics of diabetes and obesity continue to threaten the health of Americans CDC says. Press release. http://www.cdc.gov/od/oc/media/pressrel/r010911.htm
13. CDC (Centers for Disease Control and Prevention). 2002. Publications and products: National diabetes fact sheet. http://www.cdc.gov/diabetes/pubs/general.htm
14. ADA. (American Diabetes Association). 2002. Type 2 Diabetes. http://www.diabetes.org/main/application/commercewf;JSESSIONID_WLCS_DEFAULT=P Ms1ivAwuPspZ6MLBDaGp1kJ65e2IrcYW6dGivwBcCsKJ8FPPXqr!5304441 127494618142!1064251618!7501!7502?origin=*.jsp&event=link(D)
15. CDC (Centers for Disease Control and Prevention). 2001. Frequently asked questions. http://www.cdc.gov/diabetes/faqs.htm
16. CDC (Centers for Disease Control and Prevention). 2001. Diabetes: A serious public health problem at a glance 2001. http://www.cdc.gov/diabetes/pubs/glance.htm

17. NDIC (National Diabetes Information Clearinghouse). 2003. National Diabetes Statistics. http://diabetes.niddk.nih.gov/dm/pubs/statistics/index.htm
18. USCB. 2000. Historical national population estimates: July 1, 1900 to July 1, 1999. Population Division, U. S. Census Bureau. Http://www.census.gov/population/estimates/nation/popclockest.txt
19. CDC (Centers for Disease Control and Prevention). 1999. Diabetes: Impact of diabetes. http://www.cdc.gov/nccdphp/diabetes.htm
20. CDC (Centers for Disease Control and Prevention). 2002. Physician visits reach 824 million in 2000: More cardiovascular-renal, hormone and metabolic/nutrient drug visits. http://www.cdc.gov/nchs/releases/02news/physicians.htm
21. Gorman C. 2003. Why So Many of Us Are Getting Diabetes. Time Magazine. November 30. http://www.time.com/time/mqagazine/printout/0,8816,552059,00.html
22. NDIC (National Diabetes Information Clearinghouse). 2003. Diabetes Overview. http://diabetes.niddk.nih.gov/dm/pubs/overview/index.htm
23. Neergaard L. 2001. Diabetes Strikes Adults in 30's. Washington D. C. The Associated Press. August 27.
24. USDACNPP (U. S. Department of Agriculture: Center for Nutrition and Promotion). 1998. Childhood Obesity: Causes & Prevention. Symposium proceedings. October 27. http://www.usda.gov/cnpp/Seminars/obesity.PDF
25. Somer E. The Sweet Truth. 2002. http://content.health.msn.com/question_and_answer/article/1671.50536
26. CPSI (Center for Science in the Public Interest). 2000. Sugar intake hit all-time high in 1999; government urged to recommend sugar limits. Press release. http://www.cspinet.org/new/sugar_limit.html
27. DMC (DMCare). 2002. How Do Carbohydrates Affect My Blood Sugars? http://www.icsdna.com/urwhatueat/bloodcarb.html
28. Mokdad A., Ford E. S., Bowman Bxxz. A., Nelson D. E., Engelgau M. N., Vinicor F., Marks J. S. 2000. Diabetes trends in the U. S.: 1990-1998. Diabetes Care. September;23(9):1278-83.
29. DC (Diabetes Care). 2002. Screening for diabetes. Position statement. Diabetes Care. 25:S21-S24.
30. McConnaughey J. 2003. Diabetes Warning for Children. Associated Press. June 14.
31. Fredericks C. 1984. In Carlton Fredericks' New Low Blood Sugar and You. New York. Berkley Publishing.
32. BBC. (BBC News). 2002. Syndrome X the 'silent killer. April 16. http://news.bbc.co.uk/hi/english/health/newsid_1933000/1933706.stm
33. Challem J. 2000. Syndrome X. http://www.syndrome-x.com
34. Somer E. The Sweet Truth. 2002. http://content.health.msn.com/question_and_answer/article/1671.50536
35. DC (Diabetes Care). 2002. Screening for diabetes. Position statement. Diabetes Care. 25:S21-S24.
36. Day L. 2002. Attention Deficit Disorder. http://www.drday.com/attentiondeficit.htm
37. van den Berghe G., Wouters P., Weekers F., Verwaest C., Bruyninckx F., Schetz M., Vlasselaers D., Ferdinande P., Lauwers P., Bouillon R. 2001. Intensive insulin therapy in the surgical intensive care unit. New England Journal of Medicine. November;8;345(19):1417-8.

38. Benet S. 1976. In How to live to be 100. The life-style of the people of the Caucasus. P. 14-15. New York. The Dial Press.

39. Welsch C., Lachance P., Wasserman B. 1989. Dietary phenolic compounds: inhibition of Na+-dependent D-glucose uptake in rat intestinal brush border membrane vesicles. Journal of Nutrition. November;119(11):1698-704.

40. Arion W. J., Canfield W. K., Ramos F. C., Schindler P. W., Burger H. J., Hemmerle H., Schubert G., Below P., Herling A. W. 1997. Chlorogenic acid and hydroxynitrobenzaldehyde: new inhibitors of hepatic glucose 6-phosphatase. Archives of Biochemistry and Biophysics. 15; 339 (2):315-22.

41. Hemmerle H., Burger H. J., Below P., Schubert G. 1997. Chlorogenic acid and synthetic chlorogenic acid derivatives: novel inhibitors of hepatic glucose-6-phosphate translocase. The Journal of Medical Chemistry. January17;40(2):137-145.

42. Arion W. J., Canfield W. K., Ramos F. C., Schindler P. W., Burger H. J., Hemmerle H., Schubert G., Below P., Herling A. W. 1997. Chlorogenic acid and hydroxynitrobenzaldehyde: new inhibitors of hepatic glucose 6-phosphatase. Archives of Biochemistry and Biophysics. 15; 339 (2):315-22.

43. Herling A, Burger H, Schwab D., Hemmerle H, Below P, Schubert G. 1998. Pharmacodynamic profile of a novel inhibitor of the hepatic glucose-6-phosphatase system. American Journal of Physiology. June;274(6 Pt 1):G1087-93.

44. Cheng J. T., and Liu I. M. 2000. Stimulatory effect of caffeic acid on alpha1A-adrenoceptors to increase glucose uptake into cultured C2C12 cells. Naunyn-Schmiedebergs Archives of Pharmacology. 362 (2): 122-7.

45. Hsu F. L., Chen Y. C., Cheng J. T. 2000. Caffeic acid as active principle from the fruit of Xanthiumstrumarium to lower plasma glucose in diabetic rats. Planta Medica. 66(3):228-30.

46. Simon C., Herling A. W., Preibisch G, Burger H. J. 2000. Upregulation of hepatic glucose 6-phosphatase gene expression in rats treated with an inhibitor of glucose-6-phosphate translocase. Archives of Biochemistry and Biophysics. January 15;373.

47. Cignarella A., Nastasi M., Cavalli E., Puglisi L. 1996. Novel lipid-lowering properties of Vaccinium myrtillus L. leaves, a traditional antidiabetic treatment, in several models of rat dyslipidaemia: a comparison with ciprofibrate. Thrombosis Research. December1;84(5):311-22.

48. EWC (Endocrineweb.com). 2002. Normal Regulation of Blood Glucose. The Important Roles of Insulin and Glucagon: Diabetes and Hypoglycemia. http://www.endocrineweb.com/insulin.html

49. EWC (Endocrineweb.com). 2002. Diagnosing Diabetes. The Two Primary Tests and Their Results Which Combine to Make the Diagnosing of Diabetes. http://www.endocrineweb.com/diabetes/diagnosis.html

50. HFHS (Henry Ford Health System and ADAM, Inc.). 2004. Health Encyclopedia: Medical Test-Glucose Test. http://www.henryfordhealth.org/body.cfm?id=39639&action=detail&AEProductID=AdamEncy&AEArticleID=3482

51. AHA (American Heart Association). 2002. 2002 heart and stroke statistical update. http://www.americanheart.org/presenter.jhtml?identifier=3000090

52. AHA (American Heart Association). 2002. Cardiovascular disease statistics. http://216.185.112.5/presenter.jhtml?identifier=4478

53. AHA (American Heart Association). 2002. Cardiovascular disease cost. http://216.185.112.5/presenter.jhtml?identifier=4475

54. CDC (Centers for Disease Control and Prevention). 2003. Preventing Heart Disease and Stroke. http://www.cdc.gov/nccdphp/bb_heartdisease/index.htm

55. Blossom G. B. and Stephenson L. W. 1997. Heart Disease. The Grolier Multimedia Encyclopedia. Grolier Interactive, Inc.

56. Fodor J. G. and LeGrand C. 1999. Homocysteine: A new coronary heart disease risk factor. CRC (Canadian Association of Cardiac Rehabilitation) Newsletter. Fall. http://www.cacr.ca/news/1999/9909fodor.htm

57. Espinola-Klein C., Rupprecht J. J., Blankenberg S., Bickel C., Kpoo H., Rippin G., Victor A., Hafner G., Schlumberger W., Meyer J. 2002. Impact of infectious burden on extent and long-term prognosis of atherosclerosis. Circulation. January 1;105(1):15-21.

58. Kimball J. 2001. Cholesterol. http://www.ultranet.com/~jkimball/Biology/Pages/C/Cholesterol.html

59. Marieb E. N. 1995. In Human Anatomy and Physiology. Redwood City, California. The Benjamin/Cummings Publishing Company, Inc. P. 879-880.

60. Tortora G. and Anagnostakos N. 1990. In Principles of Anatomy and Physiology. New York: Biological Sciences Textbooks, Inc., A & P Textbooks, Inc., and Elia-Sparta, Inc., Harper Collins Publishers. Pp. 596 - 597.

61. Fulco A. J. 1997. Cholesterol. The Grolier Multimedia Encylopedia. Grolier Interactive, Inc

62. NIH (National Institutes of Health). 1993. So You Have High Blood Cholesterol. NIH Publication No. 93-2922.

63. Mathews C., van Holde K.. E., Ahern K. 2000. Mathews/van Holde/Ahern 3rd Edition. Foam cells. http://www.aw.com/mathews/ch18/foamcell.htm

64. SW (Science Week) 1999. Biology of Atherosclerosis. April 16. http://science-week.com/search/quajush.htm

65. Yla-Herttuala S., Palinski W., Rosenfeld M. E., Parthasarathy S., Carew T., Butler S., Witztum J. L. Steinberg D. 1989. Evidence for the presence of oxidatively modified low density lipoprotein in artherosclerotic lesions of rabbit and man. Journal of Clinical Investigation. October;84(4):1086-95

66. Steinburg D. 1990. The cholesterol controversy is over. Why did it take so long? Circulation. October;80(4):1070-8.

67. WitztumJ. L. and Steinberg D. 1991. Role of oxidized low density lipoprotein in atherogenesis. Journal of Clinical Investigation. December;88(6):1785-92. Steinbrecher U. P. 1991. Role of lipoprotein peroxidation in the pathogenesis of atherosclerosis. Clinical Cardiology. November;14(11):865-7.

68. Parthasarathy S., Printz D. J., Boyd D., Joy L., Steinberg D. 1986. Macrophage oxidation of low density lipoprotein generates a modified form recognized by the scavenger receptor. Artheriosclerosis. September-October;6950:505-10

69. Aviram M. and Fuhrman B. 1998. Polyphenolic flavonoids inhibit macrophage-mediated oxidation of LDL and attenuate atherogenesis. Atherosclerosis. 137 Suppl:S45-50.

70. Aviram M and Fuhrman B. 1998. LDL oxidation by arterial wall macrophages depends on the oxidative status in the lipoprotein and in the cells: role of prooxidants vs. antioxidants. Molecular and Cellular Biochemistry. November;188(1-2):149-59.

71. Steinbrecher U. P. 1991. Role of lipoprotein peroxidation in the pathogenesis of atherosclerosis. Clinical Cardiology. November;14(11):865-7.
72. Parthasarathy S., Printz D. J., Boyd D., Joy L., Steinberg D. 1986. Macrophage oxidation of low density lipoprotein generates a modified form recognized by the scavenger receptor. Artheriosclerosis. September-October;6950:505-10.
73. Aviram M. and Fuhrman B. 1998. Polyphenolic flavonoids inhibit macrophage-mediated oxidation of LDL and attenuate atherogenesis. Atherosclerosis. 137 Suppl:S45-50.
74. Aviram M and Fuhrman B. 1998. LDL oxidation by arterial wall macrophages depends on the oxidative status in the lipoprotein and in the cells: role of prooxidants vs. antioxidants. Molecular and Cellular Biochemistry. November;188(1-2):149-59.
75. Aviram M., Rosenblat M., Bisgaier C. L., Newton R. S., Primo-Parmo S. L., La Du B. N. 1998. Paraoxonase inhibits high-density lipoprotein oxidation and pre-serves its functions. A possible peroxidative role for paraoxonase. The Journal of Clinical Investigation. 15;101(8):1581-90.
76. Aviram M. 1999. Cholesterol oxidation, macrophage foam cells and atherosclerosis: importance of antioxidants and paraoxonase. Harefuah. 15;136(8): 620-6.
77. Cornicelli J. A., and Trivedi B. K. 1999. 15-lipoxygenase and its inhibition: A novel therapeutic target for vascular disease. Current Pharmaceutical Design. 5:11-12.
78. Smith M. L. 2002. Telephone interview of Marjorie Smith, M. D., by the author, Shaffer Fox. August 9.
79. Ross R. 1999. Atherosclerosis – an inflammatory disease. New England Journal of Medicine. January14;340(2):115-26.
80. Austin M., McKnight B., Edwards K., Bradley C., McNeely M., Psaty B., Brunzell J., Motulsky A. 2000. Cardiovascular disease mortality in familial forms of hyper-triglyceridemia: a 20-year prospective study. Circulation. 101:2777-2782.
81. MHCS (Methodist Health Care System). 2002. Pancreatitis. http://www.methodisthealth.com/endocrin/pancreat.htm
82. Coviello F. and Fuegel L. 2001. Telephone interviews of Linda Fuegel, M. T., con-sulting with Frank Coviello, by the author, Shaffer Fox, followed by written correspondence. September.
83. AHA (American Heart Association). 2002. Cholesterol statistics. http://216.185.112.5/presenter.jhtml?identifier=4506
84. AHA (American Heart Association). 2002. Cholesterol Levels. http://216.185.112.5/presenter.jhtml?identifier=4500
85. ATP III (Adult Treatment Panel III). 2001. Executive summary of the third report of the National Cholesterol Education Program (NCEP) expert panel on detection, evaluation, and treatment of high blood cholesterol in adults (adult treatment panel III). Journal of the American Medical Association. May 16;16285:19;2487-93.
86. Mortensen S. A., Leth A., Agner E., Rohde M. 1997. Dose-related decrease of serum coenzyme Q10 during treatment with HMG-CoA reductase inhibitors. Molecular Aspects of Medicine. 18 Suppl: S137-44.
87. Human J. A., Ubbink J. B., Jerling J. J., Delport R., Vermaak W. J., Vorster H. H., Lagendijk J., Potgieter H. C. 1997. The effect of Simvastatin on the plasma antioxidant concentrations in patients with hypercholesterolaemia. Clinical Chimica Acta; International Journal of Clinical Chemistry. July 4; 263(1):67-77.

88. Folkers K., Langsjoen P., Willis R., Richardson P., Xia L. J., Ye C. Q., Tamagawa H. 1990. Lovastatin decreases coenzyme Q levels in humans. Proceeding of the National Academy of Sciences of the United States of America. 87(22):8931-4.

89. Willis R. A., Folkers K., Tucker J. L., Ye C. Q., Xia L. J., Tamagawa H. 1990. Lovastatin decreases coenzyme Q levels in rats. Proceedings of the National Academy of Sciences of the United States of America. November;87(22)8928-30.

90. Palomaki A., Malminiemi K., Metsa-Ketela T. 1997. Enhanced oxidizability of ubiquinol and alpha-tocopherol during lovastatin treatment. FEBS Letters. June30;410(2-3):254-8.

91. Bhuiyan J. and Seccombe D. 1996. The effects of 3-hydroxy-3methylglutaryl-CoA reductase inhibition on tissue levels of carnitine and carnitine acyltransferase activity in the rabbit. Lipids. 31(8):867-70.

92. Kim Dong-Wook, Bang Kyu-Ho, Roh Sung-Bae, Park Won-Hwan, Kim Cheorl-Ho. 2001. Inhibitory effect of chlorogenic acid on LDL oxidation and foam cell formation. Poster Session. The Biochemical Society of the Republic of Korea. October 18.

93. Abu-Amsha R., Croft K. D., Puddley I. B., Proudfoot J. M. Beilin L. 1996. Phenolic content of various beverages determines the extent of inhibition of human serum and low-density lipoprotein oxidation in vitro: identification and mechanism of action of some cinnamic acid derivatives from red wine. Clinical Science (London). October;91(4):449-58.

94. Vieira O., Escargueil-Blanc I., Meilhac O., Basile J. P., Laranjinha J., Almeida L., Salvayre R., Negre-Salvayre A. 1998. Effect of dietary phenolic compounds on apoptosis of human cultured endothelial cells induced by oxidized LDL. British Journal of Pharmacology; 123(3):565-573.

95. Nardini M., D'Aquino M., Tomassi G., Gentili V., Di Felice M., Scaccini C. 1995. Inhibition of human low-density lipoprotein oxidation by caffeic acid and other hydroxycinnamic acid derivatives. Free Radical Biology & Medicine. 19(5):541-52.

96. Nardini M., Natella F., Gentili V., Di Felice M., Scaccini C. 1997. Effect of caffeic acid dietary supplementation on the antioxidant defense system in rat: an in vivo study. Archives of Biochemistry and Biophysics. 1; 342(1):157-160.

97. Kooy N. W., Lewis S. J., Royall J. A., Ye Y. Z., Kelly D. R., Beckman J. S. 1997. Extensive tyrosine nitration in human myocardial inflammation: evidence for the presence of peroxynitrite. Critical Care Medicine. 25(5):812-9.

98. Birks E. J. and Yocoub M. H. 1997. The role of nitric oxide and cytokines in heart failure. Coronary Artery Disease. June;8(6):389-402.

99. Beckman J. S. and Koppenol W. H. 1996. Nitric oxide, superoxide, and peroxynitrite: the good, the bad, and ugly. American Journal of Physiology. November;271(5 Pt 1):C1424-37.

100. Cross A. H., Manning P. T., Keeling R. M., Schmidt R. E., Misko T. P. 1998. Peroxynitrite formation within the central nervous system in active multiple sclerosis. Journal of Neuroimmunology. August1;88(1-2):45-56.

101. Boveris A., Valdez L. Alvarez S. 2002. Inhibition by wine pholyphenols of peroxynitrite-initiated chemiluminescence and NADA oxidation. Annals of the New York Academy of Science. May;957:90-102.

102. Pannala A. S., Razaq R., Halliwell B., Singh S., Rice-Evans C. A. 1998. Inhibition

of peroxynitrite dependent tyrosine nitration by hydroxycinnamates: nitration or electron donation? Free Radical Biology & Medicine. March 1;24(4):594-606.

103. Kono Y., Kobayashi K., Tagawa S., Adachi K., Ueda A., Sawa Y., Shibata H. 1997. Antioxidant activity of polyphenolics in diets. Rate constants of reactions of chlorogenic acid and caffeic acid with reactive species of oxygen and nitrogen. Biochimica et Biophysica Acta. June 6;1335(3):335-42.

104. NPF (National Parkinson Foundation). 2002. What the patient should know. http://www.parkinson.orgpdedu.htm

105. PAN (Parkinson's Action Network). 2001. About parkinson's disease. http://www.parkinsonaction.org

106. PAN (Parkinson's Action Network). 2003. Mission Statement. http://parkinson-action.org/aboutpan/missionstatement.htm

107. SMMMC (Saint Mary's Mercy Medical Center) and NPA (National Parkinson's Alliance. 2003. Parkinson's Disease Facts. http://www.smmmc.org/clinicalser-vices/parkinsons/facts.shtml

108. Tortora G. and Anagnostakos N. 1990. In Principles of Anatomy and Physiology. New York: Biological Sciences Textbooks, Inc., A & P Textbooks, Inc., and Elia-Sparta, Inc., Harper Collins Publishers. P. 416

109. Schapira A. H. V. 1999. Science, medicine, and the future: Parkinson's disease. The British Medical Journal. 318:311-314.

110. Kerry N., and Rice-Evans C. 1999. Inhibition of peroxynitrite-mediated oxidation of Dopamine by flavonoid and phenolic antioxidants and their structural relationships. The Journal of Neuroscience. July;73(1):247-253.

111. Manev H. and Uz Tolga. 2003. The eiscosanoid pathway and brain aging. Advances in Cell Aging and Gerontology. 12:117-136.

112. Manev H. 2003. Telephone interviews of Hari Manev, Ph.D., by the author, Shaffer Fox. July 15.

113. Uz T., Pesold C., Longone P., Manev H. 1998. Aging-associated up-regulation of neuronal 5-lipoxygenase expression: putative role in neuronal vulnerability. Journal ASEB 12(6):439-449.

114. Schafer F. Q., Yue Qian S., Buettern G. R. 2000. Iron and free radical oxidations in cell membranes. Cellular and Molecular Biology. 43(3):657-662.

115. Keller J. N., Hanni K. B., Markesbery W. R. 1999. Oxidized low-density lipoprotein induces neuronal death: implications for calcium, reactive oxygen species, and caspases. Journal of Neurochemistry. June;72(6):2601-9.

116. Sugawa M., Ikeda S., Kushima Y., Takashima Y., Cynshi O. 1997. Oxidized low density lipoprotein caused CNS neuron cell death. Brain Research. June27;761(1):165-72.

117. Schroeter H., Williams R. J., Matin R., Iversen L., Rice-Evans C. A. 2000. Phenolic antioxidants attenuate neuronal cell death following uptake of oxidized low-density lipoprotein. Free Radical Biology and Medicine. December 15;29(12):1222-33.

118. Bailey G. S., Scanlan R. A., Selivonchick D. P., Williams D. E. 1991. Food toxicology. Encyclopedia of Human Biology, ed. R. Dulbecco, Vol. 3: Pp. 671-681. New York.: Academic Press.

119. Bailey G. S. and Williams D. E. 1993. A scientific status summary by the Institute of Food Technologists'; Expert panel on food safety & nutrition. Food Technology. February;47(2):105-118.

120. BAF (Brain Aneurysm Foundation). 2003. Brain Aneurysm Basics –
Subarachnoid Hemorrhage: Fluid Buildup in the Brain.
http://www.bafound.org/subarachnoidhemorrhage.htm
121. UMM (University of Maryland Medicine). 2001. Brain Tumors: Primary –
IMMC. What Are Treatments for Some Complications of Brain tumors?
122. HCO (Heart Center Online). 2003. High-altitude Lung Ailment Examined in
Study. http://www.heartcenteronline.com/myheartdr/home/research-
detail.cfm?reutersid=2582
123. Hotchkiss J. H. 1989. Relative exposure to nitrite, nitrate, and N-nitroso compounds from endogenous and exogenous sources. In Food Toxicology, A
Perspective on the Relative Risks, ed. S. L. Taylor and R. A. Scanlan. Pp. 57-
100. New York. Marcel Dekker, Inc.
124. Peters J., Preston-Martin S., London S., Bowman J., Buckley J., Thomas D. 1994.
Precessed meats and risk of childhood leukemia. Cancer Causes Control.
Mar;5(2):195-202.
125. Cassens, R. 1997. Composition and safety of cured meats in the U. S. A. Food
Chemistry. 59:561-566.
126. Campbell M., Dunn D., Donald J., Morgan J., Golub M., Zeise L., Alexeeff G.
2000. Evidence on developmental and reproductive toxicity of sodium nitrite.
Draft document for the Reproductive and Cancer Hazard Assessment
Section, Office of Environmental Health Hazard Assessment, California
Environmental Protection Agency.
127. Hecht S. S., and Hoffman D. 1988. Tobacco-specific nitrosamines, an important
group of carcinogens in tobacco and tobacco smoke. Carcinogenesis. 9:875-884.
128. NAS (National Academy of Sciences). 1981. The health effects of nitrate,
nitrite and N-nitroso compounds. Washington, D. C. National Academy Press.
129. Kono Y., Shibata H., Kodama Y., Sawa Y. 1995. The suppression of the N-
nitrosating reaction by chlorogenic acid. The Biochemical Journal.
Devember15;312 (Pt3):947-953.
130. Kono Y., Shibata H., Kodama Y., Ueda A., Sawa Y. 1995. Chlorogenic acid as a
natural scavenger for hypochlorous acid. Biochemical and Biophysical
Research Communications. 217(3):972-8.
131. Shimizu M., Yoshimi N., Yamada Y., Matsunaga K., Kawabata K., Hara A.,
Moriwaki H., Mori H. 1999. Suppressive effects of chlorogenic acid on N-
methyl-N-nitrosourea-induced glandular stomach carcinogenesis in male
F344 rats. The Journal of Toxicological Sciences. 24(5):433-9.
132. Mori H , Tanaka T., Shima H., Kuniyasu T., Takahashi M. 1986. Inhibitory effect
of chlorogenic acid on methylazoxymethanol acetate-induced carcinogenesis
in large intestine and liver of hamsters. Cancer Letters. 30 (1):49-54.
133. Kasai H., Fukada S., Yamaizumi Z., Sugie S., Mori H. 2000. Action of chlorogenic acid in vegetables and fruits as an inhibitor of 8-hydroxydeoxyguano-
sine formation in vitro and in a rat carcinogenesis model. Food and Chemical
Toxicology. 38(5):467-471.
134. Whalen M. M. and Loganathan B. G. 2001. Butyltin exposure causes a rapid
decrease in cyclic AMP levels in human lymphocytes. Toxicology and Applied
Pharmacology. March 15; 171(3):141-8.
135. Whalen M. M., Ghazi S., Loganathan B. G., Hatcher F. 2002. Expression of
CD16, CD18 and CD56 in tributyltin-exposed human natural killer cells.
Chemico-Biological Interactions. February 20;139(2):159-76

136. Fox M. 2002. Pesticide exposure suppresses the human immune system. Reuters. April 10. Biodiversity & Human Health. http://www.wms.org/biod/habitat/news/Phenyltins.html

137. Fox M. 2002. Pesticide combination leads to Parkinson's. Reuters. January 4.

138. Brasher P. 2002. Study finds pesticides in some organic food. Associated Press. May 8.

139. Saleh A., Faten N., Ayyash O., Gasteyer S. 1995. Pesticide usage in the West Bank. Report for the Applied Research Institute-Jerusalem (ARIJ).

140. PN (Pesticides News). 1996. Pesticides News. Paraquat fact sheet. Journal of the Pesticides Trust. June(32).

141. TPH (Toronto Public Health). 1998. Pesticides: A Public Health Perspective. Technical Report. Environmental Protection Office. P. 15.

142. Fisher B. E. 1999. Radically new research. Environmental Health Perspectives. February;107(2). http://ehpnet1.niehs.nih.gov/docs/1999/107-2/niehsnews.html

143. Dekker J. 1997. Paraquat. http://www.agron.iastate.edu/~weeds/Ag317/manage/herbicide/paraquat.html

144. Thomas C. E. and Aust S. D. Reductive release of iron from ferritin by cantion free radicals of paraquat and other bipyridyls. The Journal of Biological Chemistry. October5;261(28):13064-70.

145. Buettner G. R. and Schafer F. Q. 2000. Free radicals, oxidants, and antioxidants. Teratology 62:234

146. Tsuchiya T., Suzuki O., Igarashi K. 1996. Protective effects of chlorogenic acid on paraquat-induced oxidative stress in rats. Bioscience, Biotechnology, and Biochemistry. 60(5):765-8.

147. Skalinder L. E. 1999. Radiation. Compton's Interactive Encyclopedia.

148. Griffiths A. J. F. 1997. Genetics. The Grolier Multimedia Encylopedia. Grolier Interactive, Inc.

149. Kohlein W. 1997. The Effects of Alpha-Particles on Chromosomal Alterations. http://www.foe.arc.net.au/kohnlein/kohnpaper4.html

150. NSBRI (National Space Flight Research Institute). 2003. Radiation and Long-Term Space Flight. http://www.nsbri.org/Radiation/HumanAffects.html

151. Skalinder L. E. 1999. Radiation. Compton's Interactive Encyclopedia.

152. Gofman J. W. 2001. X-Radiation and Gamma Radiation: Comments on Their Nomination as Known Human Carcinogens for the Eleventh Report on Carcinogens (RoC). http://www.ratical.org/radiation/CNR/XHP/NTP.html

153. Bondy M. L., Wang L. E., El-Zein R., de Andrade M., Selvan M. S., Bruner J. M., Levin V. A., Alfred Yung W. K., Adatto P., Wei Q. 2001. Gamma-radiation sensitivity and risk of glioma. Journal of the National Cancer Institute. October 17;93(20):1553-7.

154. Abraham S. K., Sarma L., Kesavan P. C. 1993. Protective effects of chlorogenic acid, curcumin and beta- carotene against gamma-radiation-induced in vivo chromosomal damage. Mutation Research. 303 (3): 109-12.

155. Sedano H. O. 1998. Oral Herpes Simplex Infections. http://www.dent.ucla.edu/ftp/pic/visitors/herpes/page1.html

156. Cooper G. G. 2000. HSV-1,HSV-2. http://www.brown.edu/Courses/Bio_160/Projects2000/Herpes/HSV/home.html

157. Emory (Emory University Health Sciences News and Information). 1997. One in five Americans infected with genital herpes: prevalence has increased 30

percent in past 20 years; greatest increase in white teens, says CDC/Emory team in NEJM. October 19. http://www.emory.edu/WHSC/HSNEWS/releases/oct97/herpes_namias.html

158. CDC (Centers for Disease Control and Prevention). 2002. Tracking the hidden epidemics 2000. Trends in STDs in the United States. Trends by disease. Herpes. December 4. http://www.dcd.gov/nchstp/od/news/RevBrochure1pdfHerpes.htm

159. Absalon J. 2003. Sexually Transmitted Diseases. http://www.columbia.edu/~am430/std.htm

160. Fisman D. N., Lipsitch M., Hook E. W. III., Goldie S. J. 2002. Projection of the future dimensions and costs of the genital herpes simplex type 3 epidemic in the United States. Sexually Transmitted Diseases. October;29(10):608-22.

161. SD (Science Daily Magazine). 2000. New evidence found linking herpes and Alzheimer's. May 12. http://www.sciencedaily.com/releases/2000/05/000512083302.htm

162. Pyles R. B. 2001. The association of herpes simplex virus and Alzheimer's Disease: a potential synthesis of genetic and environmental factors. Herpes. November;8(3):64-8.

163. Al Wattar N. 2002. The relationship between inflammation and heart disease. http://www.arabmedmag.com/general/egeneralinfo04.htm

164. ACS (American Cancer Society). 2002. Infectious agents and cancer. http://www.cancer.org/eprise/main/docroot/PED/content/PED_1_3X_Infectious_Agents_and_Cancer?sitearea=PED

165. Dwyer D. E. and Cunningham A. L. 2002. 10: Herpes simplex and varicella-zoster virus infections. MJA practice essentials – Infectious diseases. The Medical Journal of Australia. 177(5):267-273.

166. Sedano H. O. 1998. Oral Herpes Simplex Infections. http://www.dent.ucla.edu/ftp/pic/visitors/herpes/page1.html

167. Thiel K. D., Helbig B., Klocking R., Wutzler P., Sprossig M., Schweizer H. 1981. Comparison of the in vitro activities of ammonium humate and of enzymically oxidized chlorogenic and caffeic acids against type 1 and type 2 human herpes virus. Pharmazie. 36(1):50-3.

168. Binutu O. A., Adesogan K. E., Okogun J. I. 1996. Antibacterial and antifungal compounds from Kigelia pinnata. Planta Medica. August;62(4):352-3.

169. Cai L., and Wu C. D. 1996. Compounds from Syzygium aromaticum possessing growth inhibitory activity against oral pathogens. Journal of Natural Products. 59(10):987-90.

170. Aziz N. H., Farag S. E., Mousa L. A., Abo-Zaid M. A. 1998. Comparative antibacterial and antifungal effects of some phenolic compounds. Microbios. 93(374):43-54.

171. Barber M. S., McConnell V. S., DeCaux B. S. 2000. Antimicrobial intermediates of the general phenylpropanoid and ligin specific pathways. Phytochemistry. May;54(1):53-6.

172. Velikova M., Bankova V., Sorkun K., Houcine S., Tsvetkova I., Kujumgiev A. 2000. Propolis from the Mediterranean region: chemical composition and antimicrobial activity. Zeitschrift für Naturforschung. September-October;55(9-10):790-3.

173. Chiang L. C., Chiang W., Chang M. Y., Ng L. T., Lin C. C. 2002. Antiviral activity of Plantago major extracts and related compounds in vitro. Antiviral

Research. July;55(1):53-62.
174. AP (The Associated Press). 2002. U. N. warns of HIV/AIDS spread. July 2.
http://abcnews.go.com/wire/World/ap200020702_702.html
175. Rigby B. 2002. AIDS epidemic surges, 70 million may die, U. N. says. Reuters.
July 2.
176. Susman E. 2002. Report: 40 million living with AIDS.
http://www.upi.com/view.cfm?StoryID=02072002-071823-5080r
177. CDC (Centers for Disease Control and Prevention). 2002. Living with AIDS.
http://www.cdc.gov/hiv/pubs/brochure/livingwithhiv.htm
178. Kreis W., Kaplan M. H., Freeman J., Sun D. K., Sarin P. S. 1990. Inhibition of
HIV replication by Hyssop officinalis extracts. Antiviral Research.
December;14(6):323-37.
179. Robinson W. E., Reinecke M. G., Abdel-Malek S., Jia Q., Chow S. A. 1996.
Inhibitors of HIV-1 replication [corrected; erratum to be published] that
inhibit integrase. Proceedings of the National Academy of Sciences of the
United States of America. June25;93(13):6326-31.
180. Robinson W. E., Cordeiro M., Abdel-Malek S., Jia Q., Chow S., Reinecke M.,
Mitchell W. M. 1996. Dicaffeoylquinic acid inhibitors of human immunodeficiency virus integrase: inhibition of the core catalytic domain of human
immunodeficiency virus integrase. Molecular Pharmacology. October;50(4):
846-55.
181. McDougall B., King P. J., Wu B. W., Hostomsky Z., Reinecke M. G., Robinson
W. E., Jr. 1998. Dicaffeoylquinic and dicaffeoyltartaric acids are selective
inhibitors of human immunodeficiency virus type 1 intergrase. Antimicrobial
Agents and Chemotherapy. January;42(1):140-6.
182. Zhu K., Cordeiro M. L., Atienza J., Robinson W. E., Chow S. A. 1999.
Irreversible inhibition of human immunodeficiency virus type 1 integrase by
dicaffeoylquinic acids. Journal of Virology. April;73(4):3309-16.

CHAPTER 5. GEORGIAN POMEGRANATE

1. Grieve M. 1995. A modern herbal: Pomegranate.
http://www.botanical.com/botanical/mgmh/p/pomegr60.html
2. BSP (Branch -Smith Publishing). 1999. Punica granatum. http://www.green-
beam.com/features/plant041299.stm
3. Felter H. W. and Lloyd J. U. 1898. Granatum (U. S. P.) – Pomegranate. In King's
American Dispensatory. http://www.ibiblio.org/herbmed/eclectic/kings/puni-
ca.html
4. Knight R. J., Jr. 1997. Pomegranate. The Grolier Multimedia Encyclopedia. Grolier
Interactive, Inc.
5. Lloyd J. U. 1897. Punica Granatum. The Western Druggist. May.
6. Winer B. 1961. In The Ancient World. New York. Random House. Pp. 112-113.
7. (UK) Unknown Jewish Captive of Babylon (560-538 B. C.). 1977. In The New
American Standard Bible. Nashville. Thomas Nelson Publishers. 1st Kings VII,
18, 20.
8. Moses. (1446 - 1290 B. C.). 1977. In The New American Standard Bible.
Nashville. Thomas Nelson Publishers. Exodus XXVIII, 33, 34.

9. Moses. (1446 B. C. -). 1977. In The New American Standard Bible. Nashville. Thomas Nelson Publishers. Deuteronomy 8:8.
10. Ross A. S. 2002. Peirot Eretz Yisrael/Birchat Me'eyn Shalosh. Introduction. http://pages.nyu.edu/~asr209/peirot.html
11. Ramazanov Z. 2000. Data provided to the author, Shaffer Fox.
12. IME (The Israel Museum Exhibit). 2002. Ivory pomegranate. http://www.imj.org.il/archaeology/ivory.htm
13. Janick J. 2002. History of horticulture. Lectures 23-24. Herbals: The connection between horticulture and medicine. http://www.hort.purdue.edu/newcrop/history/lecture23/lec231.html
14. Kemertelidze E. P. 2003. Telephone interview of E. P. Kemertelidze, D.Sc., by the author, Shaffer Fox. July 24.
15. Felter H. W. 1922. In The Eclectic Materia Medica, Pharmacology and Therapeutics. Cincinnati. John K. Scudder. P. 206-7.
16. Ben Nasr C., Ayed N., Metche M. 1996. Quantitative determination of the polyphenolic content of pomegranate peel. Zeitschrift fur Lebensmittel-untersuchung und - forchung. 203(4):374-8.18.
17. Moneam N. M., el Sharaky A. S., Badreldin M. M. 1988. Estrogen content of pomegranate seeds. J Chromatogr 22; 438(2): 438-42.
18. ACS (American Cancer Society). 2002. Cancer Facts & Figures 2002. http://www.cancer.org/downloads/STT/Cancerpercent20Factspercent20&per-cent20Figurespercent202002percent20RevCovP6P7TmPWSecured.pdf
19. ACS (American Cancer Society). 2003. Cancer Facts & Figures 2003. http://www.cancer.org/downloads/STT/CAFF2003PWSecured.pdf
20. NYSDH (New York State Department of Health). 1999. Chronic disease teaching tools - about cancer. http://www.health.state.ny.us/nysdoh/chronic/aboutc.htm
21. Rich W. M. 2002. What is cancer? http://www.gyncancer.com/what-is.html
22. O'Connell D. 2002. Telephone interview of Daniel O'Connell, Ph.D., by the author, Shaffer Fox, for the purpose of a third party accuracy review of the paragraph cited. June 24.
23. Pitot H. C. 1997. Cancer (disease). The Grolier Multimedia Encyclopedia. Grolier Interactive, Inc.
24. Rich W. M. 2002. Telephone interview of William M. Rich, M. D., by the author, Shaffer Fox. June 24.
25. Moss M. 2002. Spotting breast cancer: doctors are weak link. The New York Times. June 27.
26. Morowitz H. 1997. Cell. The Grolier Multimedia Encyclopedia. Grolier Interactive, Inc.
27. MHCS (Methodist Health Care System). 2002. Cancer. http://www.methodisthealth.com/cancer/index.htm
28. Kaku M. 1997. In Visions: How Science Will Revolutionize the 21st Century. New York. Anchor Books. P. 166.
29. Festa F., Aglitti T., Duranti G., Ricordy R., Perticone P., Cozzi R. 2001. Strong antioxidant activity of ellagic acid in mammalian cells in vitro revealed by the comet assay. Anticancer Research. November - December;21(6A):3903-8.
30. Medem (Medem, Inc.). 2000. Cancer basics: What is cancer? http://www.medem.com/MedLB/article_detaillb.cfm?article_ID=zzzz6I0LZ6C&sub_cat=260

31. Tortora G. and Anagnostakos N. 1990. In Principles of Anatomy and Physiology. New York: Biological Sciences Textbooks, Inc., A & P Textbooks, Inc., and Elia-Sparta, Inc., Harper Collins Publishers. P. 84

32. Bhattacharya S. 2003. Study Reveals Chemical Cocktail in Every Person. NewScientist.com News Service. November 3. http://www.newscientist.com/news/print.jsp?id=99994414

33. WWF (World Wildlife Federation). 2003. National Biomonitoring Survey 2003. http://www.wwf-uk.org/filelibrary/pdf/biomonitoringresults.pdf

34. Carpenter D. O. 2001. Studies Link PCB's to Human Cancer. Wall Street Journal. January 4. Editorial page commentary. http://www.minfully.org/Pesticide/PCBs-Human-Cancer.htm

35. USEPA (United States Environmental Protection Agency). 2002. Health Effects of PCBs. http://www.epa.gov/opptintr/pcb/effects.html

36. NJDHSS (New Jersey Department of Health and Senior Services). 1996. Hazardous Substance Fact Sheet: DICHLORVOS. http://www.state.nj.us/health/eoh/rtkweb/0674.pdf

37. WHO (World Health Organization). 2003. WHO and FAO Announce a Unified Approach To Promote Fruit and Vegetable Consumption. http://www.who.int/hpr/

38. Jiang Y., Kusama K., Satoh K., Takayama E., Watanabe S., Sakagami H. 2000. Induction of cytotoxicity by chlorogenic acid in human oral tumor cell lines. Phytomedicine. December;7(6):483-91.

39. Jiang Y., Satoh K., Watanabe S., Kusama K., Sakagami H. 2001. Inhibition of chlorogenic-induced cytotoxicity by CoC12. Anticancer Research. September - October;21(5):3349-53.

40. Kaul A., and Khanduja K. L. 1998. Polyphenols inhibit promotional phase of tumorigenesis: relevance of superoxide radicals. Nutrition and Cancer. 32(2):81-5.

41. Chan W. S., Wen P. C., Chiang H. C. 1995. Structure-activity relationship of caffeic acid analogue on xanthine oxidase inhibition. Anticancer Research. May-June;15(3):703-7

42. Lesca P. 1983. Protective effects of ellagic acid and other plant phenols on benzo(a)pyrene-induced neoplasia in mice. Carcinogenesis. December;4(12):1651-1653.

43. Chang R. L., Hùang M. T., Wood A.W., Wong C. Q., Newmark H. L., Yagi H., Sayer J. M., Jerina D., Conney A. H. 1985. Effect of ellagic acid and hydroxylated flavonoids on the tumorigenicity of benzo(a)pyrene and (")-78ß,8a-dihydroxy-9a,10a-epoxy-7,8,9,10 tetrahydrobenzo(a) pyrene on mouse skin and in the newborn mouse. Carcinogenesis. August;6(8):1127-1133.

44. Boukharta M., Jalbert G., Castonguay A. 1992. Biodistribution of ellagic acid and dose-related inhibition of lung tumorigenesis in A/J mice. Nutrition and Cancer. 18(2):181-9.

45. Walton M. 2002. Mice, men share 99 percent of genes. December 4. CNN.com/Science & Space. http://www.cnn.com/2002/TECH/science/12/04/coolsc.coolsc.mousegenome

46. Mandal S., and Stoner G. D. 1990. Inhibition of N-nitrosobenzyl-methylamine-induced esophageal tumorigenesis in rats by ellagic acid. Carcinogenesis. January;11(1):55-61.

47. Siglin, J. C., Barch D., Stoner G. D. 1995. Effects of phenethyl isothiocyanate,

ellagic acid, sulindac and supplementary dietary calcium on the induction and progression of esophageal carcinogenesis in rats induced by short-term administration of N-nitrosomethylbenzylamine. Carcinogenesis. May;16(5):1101-6.

48. Daniel E. and Stoner G. 1991. The effects of ellagic acid and 13-cis-retinoic acid on N-nitrosobenzylmethylamine-induced esophagal tumorigenesis in rats. Cancer Letters. 56(2):117-24.

49. Mandal S., Ahuja A., Shivapurkar N., Cheng S., Groopman J., Stoner G. 1987. Inhibition of aflatoxin B1 mutagenesis in Salmonella typhimurium and DNA damage in cultured rat and human tracheobronchial tissues by ellagic acid. Carcinogenesis. 11: 55-61.

50. Tanaka T., Iwata H., Niwa K., Mori Y., Mori H. 1988. Inhibitory effect of ellagic acid on N-2-fluoenylacetamide-induced liver carcinogenesis in male AC1/N rats. Japanese Journal of Cancer Research: Gann. December;79:1297-303.

51. Priyadarsini K. I., Khopde S. M., Kumar S. S., Mohan H. 2002. Free radical studies of ellagic acid, a natural phenolic antioxidant. Journal of Agricultural and Food Chemistry. March 27;50(7):2200-6.

52. Tanaka T., Kojima T., Kawamori T., Wang A., Suzui M., Okamoto K., Mori H. 1993. Inhibition of 4-nitroquinoline-1-oxide-induced rat tongue carcinogenesis by the naturally occurring plant phenolics caffeic, ellagic, chlorogenic and ferulic acids. Carcinogenesis. July;14(7):1321-5.

53. Mukhtar H., Das M., Del Tito B., Bickers D. 1984. Protection against 3-methylcholanthrene-induced skin tumorigenesis in BALB/c mice by ellagic acid. Biochemical and Biophysical Research Communications. 119: 751-757.

54. Mukhtar H., Das M., Bickers D. 1986. Inhibition of 3-methylcholanthrene-induced skin tumorigenicity in BALB/c mice by chronic oral feeding of trace amounts of ellagic acid in drinking water. Cancer Research. 46: 2262-2265.

55. Gali H. U., Perchellet E. M., Klish D. S., Johnson J. M., Perchellet J. P. 1992. Hydrolyzable tannins: potent inhibitors of hydroperoxide production and tumor promotion in mouse skin treated with 12-O-tetradecanoylphorbol-13-acetate in vivo. International Journal of Cancer. May 28;51(3):425-32.

56. Ho C. C., Tsai H. Y., Lai Y. S., Chung J. G. 2001. Ellagic acid inhibited 2-aminofluorene and p-aminobenzoic acid acetylation by mononuclear leucocytes from Sprague-Dawley rats. Cytobios. 104(406):107-17.

57. Lin S. S., Hung C. F., Ho C. C., Liu Y. H., Ho H. C., Chung J. G. 2000. Effects of ellagic acid by oral administration on N-acetylation and metabolism of 2-aminofluorene in rat brain tissues. Neurochemical Research. November;25(11):1503-8.

58. Lin S. S., Hung C. F., Tyan Y. S., Yang C. C., Hsia T. C., Yang M. D., Chung J. G. 2001. Ellagic acid inhibits arylamine N-acetyltransferase activity and DNA adduct formation in human bladder tumor cell lines (T24 and TSGH 8301). Urological Research. December;29(6):371-6.

59. Nijhoff W. A. and Peters W. H. 1994. Quantification of induction of rat oesophageal, gastric and pancreatic glutathione and glutathione S-transferases by dietary anticarcinogens. Carcinogenesis. September;15(9):1769-72.

60. Narayanan B. A., Narayanan N. K., Stoner G. D., Bullock B. P. 2002. Interactive gene expression pattern in prostate cancer cells exposed to phenolic antioxidants. Life Sciences. March 1;70(15):1821-39.

61. Narayanan B. A., Re G. G. 2001. IGF-II down regulation associated cell cycle arrest in colon cancer cells exposed to phenolic antioxidant ellagic acid.

Anticancer Research. January-February;21(1A):359-64.
62. Hayatsu H., Arimoto S., Negishi T. 1998. Dietary inhibitors of mutagenesis and carcinogenesis. Mutation Research. December; 202(2):429-46.
63. Chang R. L., Hùang M. T., Wood A.W., Wong C. Q., Newmark H. L., Yagi H., Sayer J. M., Jerina D., Conney A. H. 1985. Effect of ellagic acid and hydroxylated flavonoids on the tumorigenicity of benzo(a)pyrene and (")-78ß,8a-dihydroxy-9a,10a-epoxy-7,8,9,10 tetrahydrobenzo(a) pyrene on mouse skin and in the newborn mouse. Carcinogenesis. August;6(8):1127-1133.
64. Dixit R. and Gold B. 1986. Inhibition of N-methyl-N-nitrosourea-induced mutagenicity and DNA methylation by ellagic acid. Proceedings of the National Academy of Sciences of the United States of America. 83: 8039-8043.
65. Smart R. C., Huang M. T., Chang R. L., Sayer J. M., Jerina D. M., Conney A. H. 1986. Disposition of the naturally occurring antimutagenic plant phenol, ellagic acid, and its synthetic derivatives, 3-0-decylellagic acid and 3,3'-di-0-methylellagic acid in mice. Carcinogenesis. October;7(10):1663-7.
66. Pepin P., Rossignol G., Castonguay A. 1990. Inhibition of NNK-induced lung tumorigenesis in A/J mice by ellagic acid and butylated hydroxyanisole. Cancer Journal. 3: 266-273.
67. Barch D. and Iannaccone P. 1986. Role of zinc deficiency in carcinogenesis. Advances in Experimental Medicine and Biology. 206:517-27.
68. Barch D. and Fox C. 1987. Dietary zinc deficiency increases the methylbenzylnitrosamine-induced formation of 06–methylguanine in the esophageal DNA of the rat. Carcinogenesis. October;8(10):1461-4.
69. Barch D. and Rundhaugen L 1994. Ellagic acid induces NAD (P) H: quinone reductase through activation of the antioxidant responsive element of the rat NAD (P)H: quinone reductase gene. Carcinogenesis. 15(9):2065-8.
70. ACS (American Cancer Society). 2001. Cervical cancer overview. Cancer Resource Center.
http://www3.cancer.org/cancerinfo/load_cont.asp?ct=8&doc=25&Language=English
71. ACS (American Cancer Society). 2002. Cancer Facts & Figures 2002.
http://www.cancer.org/downloads/STT/Cancerpercent20Factspercent20&percent20Figuarespercent202002percent20RevCovP6P7TmPWSecured.pdf
72. ACS (American Cancer Society) 2002. Breast Cancer Facts & Figures 2001-2002.
http://www.cancer.org/eprise/main/docroot/stt/content/STT_1x_Breast_Cancer_Facts_and_Figures_2001-2002
73. NCI (National Cancer Institute). 2001. Cancer Facts: lifetime probability of breast cancer in American women. http://cis.nci.nih.gov/fact/5_6.htm
74. ACS (American Cancer Society). 2001. What causes breast cancer? http://www.cancer.org/docroot/cri/content/cri_2_2_2xwhat_causes_breast_cancer_5.asp?sitearea=cri
75. Smith W. A. and Gupta R. C. 1996. Use of microsome-mediated test system to assess efficacy and mechanisms of cancer chemopreventive agents. Carcinogenesis. June;17(6):1285-90.
76. Smith W. A., Arif J. M., Gupta R. C. 1998. Effect of chemopreventive agents on microsome-mediated DNA adduction of the breast carcinogen dibenzo[a, l]pyrene. Mutation Research. February 13;412(3):307-14.
77. Smith W. A. and Gupta R. C. 1999. Determining efficacy of cancer chemopreventive agents using a cell-free system concomitant with DNA adduction.

Mutation Research. March 10;425(1):143-52.
78. Smith W. A., Freeman J. W., Gupta R. C. 2001. Effect of chemopreventive agents on DNA adduction induced by the potent mammary carcinogen dibenzo[a, l]pyrene in the human breast cells MCF-7. Mutation Research. September 1;480-481:97-108.
79. Smith W. A. 2001. Telephone interviews of W. A. Smith, Ph.D., by the author.
80. Kim N. D., Mehta R., Yu W., Neeman I., Livney T., Amichay A., Poirier D., Nicholls P., Kirby A., Jiang W., Mansel R., Ramachandran C., Rabi T., Kaplan B., Lansky E. 2002. Chemopreventive and adjuvant therapeutic potential of pomegranate (Punica granatum) for human breast cancer. Breast Cancer Research and Treatment. February;71(3):203-17.
81. ACS (American Cancer Society). 2001. Cervical cancer overview. Cancer Resource Center. http://www3.cancer.org/cancerinfo/load_cont.asp?ct=8&doc=25&Language= English
82. ACS (American Cancer Society). 2003. What Are the Risk Factors for Cervical Cancer. Detailed Guide: Cervical Cancer. http://www.cancer.org/docroot/CRI/content/CRI_2_4_2X_What_are_the_ris k_factors_for_cervical_cancer_8.asp?sitearea=
83. Tortora G. and Anagnostakos N. 1990. In Principles of Anatomy and Physiology. New York: Biological Sciences Textbooks, Inc., A & P Textbooks, Inc., and Elia-Sparta, Inc., Harper Collins Publishers. P. 919.
84. Cheonis N. 2001. Anal neoplasia: a growing concern. Bulletin of Experimental Treatment for Aids. Winter.
85. UMAUHS. University of Massachusetts Amherst, University Health Services). 2003. Genital Warts and HPV (human papillomavirus). http://www.umass.edu/uhs/warts.html
86. HC (Health Canada). 2003. What You Need to Know About Human Papillomavirus (HPV). http://www.hc-sc.gc.ca/pphb-dgspsp/std-mts/pdf/hpv-e.pdf
87. Herrero R, Castellsague X, Pawlita M, Lissowska J, Kee F, Balaram P, Rajkumar T, Sridhar H, Rose B, Pintos J, Fernandez L, Idris A, Sanchez MJ, Nieto A, Talamini R, Tavani A, Bosch FX, Reidel U, Snijders PJ, Meijer CJ, Viscidi R, Munoz N, Franceschi S; IARC Multicenter Oral Cancer Study Group. 2003. Human papillomavirus and oral cancer: the International Agency for Research on Cancer Multicenter study. Journal of the National Cancer Institute. December 3;95(23):1772-83.
88. Zu W. G., Zhang L. J., Lu Z. M., Li J. Y., Ke Y., Zu G. W. 2003. Detection of human papillomavirus type 16 E6 mRNA in carcinomas of upper digestive tract. Zhonghua Yi Xue Za Zhi. November 10;83(21):1910-4.
89. CDC (Centers for Disease Control and Prevention) 2001. Genital H. P. V. infection. S. T. D. prevention. Division of sexually transmitted diseases. . http://www.cdc.gov/nchstp/dstd/Fact_Sheets/FactsHPV.htm
90. NCI (National Cancer Institute). 2000. Prevention of cervical cancer – updated. National Cancer Institute/PDQ Physician Statement. OncoLink. University of Pennsylvania Cancer Center. http://cancer.med.upenn.edu/pdq_html/3/engl/304734-3.html.
91. Herrero R., Hildesheim A., Concepcion B., Sherman M., Hutchinson M., Morales J., Balmaceda I., Greenberg M., Alfaro M., Burk R., Wacholder S.,

Plummer M., Schiffman M. 2001. Population-based study of human papillomavirus infection and cervical neoplasia in rural Costa Rica. Journal of the
National Cancer Institute. March;92(6):464-74.

92. Monsonego J, Bosch FX, Coursaget P, Cox JT, Franco E, Frazer I,
Sankaranarayanan R, Schiller J, Singer A, Wright T, Kinney W, Meijer C,
Linder J. 2004. Cervical cancer control, priorities and new directions.
International Journal of Cancer. January 20;108(3):329-33.

93. Warner J. 2003. Cancer-Virus Link Growing Quickly. WebMD Medical News.
December 10.
http://wolsvc.health.webmd.aol.com/content/Article/78/95750.htm

94. Muñoz N., Bosch F. X., de Sanjosé S., Herrero R., Castellsagué X., Shah, K. V.,
Snijders P. J. F., Meijer, C. J. L. M., for the International Agency for Research
on Cancer Multicenter Cervical Cancer Study Group. 2003. Epidemiologic
classification of human papillomavirus types associated with cervical cancer.
The New England Journal of Medicine. 348:518-527.

95. Gardner A. 2003. Study Identifies Major Viruses Tied to Cervical Cancer.
HealthScoutNews. Thursday, February 6.
http://www.hon.ch/News/HSN/511639.html

96. Sasagawa T., Basha W., Yamazaki H., Inoue M. 2001. High-risk and multiple
human papillomavirus infections associated with cervical abnormalities in
Japanese women. Cancer Epidemiology Biomarkers & Prevention.
January;10:45-52.

97. Reeves W. C., Rawls W. E., Brinton L. A. 1989. Epidemiology of genital papillomaviruses and cervical cancer. Review of Infectious Disease. 11(3):426-39.

98. Narayanan A., Geoffroy O., Willingham M., Re Gian., Nixon D. 1999. p53/p21
(WAF1/CIP1) expression and its possible role in G1 arrest and apoptosis in
ellagic acid treated cancer cells. Cancer Letters. 136:215-221.

99. UPCI (University of Pittsburgh Cancer Institute). 2002. Drug slows growth of
precancerous lung lesions.
http://www.upci.upmc.edu/internet/news/reuters/reuters.cfm?article=495

100. BCCA (British Columbia Cancer Agency). 2000. Respiratory system – lung.
http://204.174.66.178/cid/20.shtml

101. BCCA (British Columbia Cancer Agency). 2002. 2002 BC Cancer Agency
News – 2002/04/09: Dry mouth agent may help prevent lung cancer.
http://www.cccancer.bc.ca/ABCCA/NewsCentre?2002BCCancerAgencyNew
s/ADTstudy.htm

102. Kidd P. M. 2002. Glutathione: Systemic protectant against oxidative and free
radical damage. http://www.thorne.com/altmedrev/fulltext/glut.html

103. Cross C. E., Halliwell B., Borish E. T., Pryor W. A., Ames B. N., Saul R. L.,
McCord J. M., Harman D. 1987. Oxygen radicals and human disease. Annals
of Internal Medicine. October;107(4):526-4595.

104. Teel R. and Castonguay A. 1992. Antimutagenic effects of polyphenolic compounds. Cancer Letters. September30;66(2):107-13.

105. Romert L., Jansson T., Curvall M., Jenssen D. 1994. Screening for agents inhibiting the mutagenicity of extracts and constituents of tobacco products.
Mutation Research. 322 (2):97-110.

106. Khanduja K. L., Gandhi R. K., Pathania V., Syal N. 1999. Prevention of N-
nitrosodiethylamine-induced lung tumorigenesis by ellagic acid and quercetin
in mice. Food and Chemical Toxicology. 37(4):313-8.

107. Kabat G. C., Ng S. K., Wynder E. L. 1993. Tobacco, alcohol intake, and diet in relation to adenocarcinoma of the esophagus and gastric cardia. Cancer Causes Control. March;4(2):123-32.
108. Stemmermann G. N., Nomura A. M., Chyou P. H., Yoshizawa C. 1990. Prospective study of alcohol intake and large bowel cancer. Digestive Diseases and Sciences. November;35(11):1414-20.
109. Iino T., Nakahara K., Miki W., Kiso Y., Ogawa Y., Kato S., Takeuchi K. 2001. Less damaging effect of whisky in rat stomachs in comparison with pure ethanol. Role of ellagic acid, the nonalcoholic component. Digestion. 64(4):214-21.
110. Iino T., Tashima K., Umeda M., Ogawa Y., Takeeda M., Takata K., Takeuchi K. 2002. Effect of ellagic acid on gastric damage induced in ischemic rat stomachs following ammonia or reperfusion. Life Sciences. January;70(10):1139-50.
111. Stumpfl M. E. and Weiner J. 2002. Polyphenols in tea may reduce risk of stomach, esophagus cancers. University of Southern California. Press release. April 8.
112. DeNoon D. 2002. Common Foods Help Prevent Cancer. April 9. http://aolsvc.health.webmd.aol.com/printing/article/2946.1057
113. Gil M., Tomas-Barberan F., Hess-Pierce B., Holcroft D., Kader A. 2000. Antioxidant activity of pomegranate juice and its relationship with phenolic composition and processing. Journal of Agricultural and Food Chemistry. Oct;48(10):4581-9.
114. Aviram M. 1993. Modified forms of low density lipoprotein and atherosclerosis. Atherosclerosis. January 4;98(1):1-9.
115. Aviram M. 1996. Interaction of oxidized low density lipoprotein with macrophage in atherosclerosis, and the antiatherogenicity of antioxidants. European Journal of Clinical Chemistry and Clinical Biochemistry. August;34(8):599-608.
116. Aviram M., Rosenblat M., Bisgaier C. L., Newton R. S., Primo-Parmo S. L., La Du B. N. 1998. Paraoxonase inhibits high-density lipoprotein oxidation and preserves its functions. A possible peroxidative role for paraoxonase. The Journal of Clinical Investigation. 15;101(8):1581-90.
117. Maor I., Hayek T., Hirsh M., Iancu T. C., Aviram M. 2000. Macrophage-released proteoglycans enhance LDL aggregation: studies in aorta from apolipoprotein E-deficient mice. Atherosclerosis. 150(1):91-101.
118. Maor I., Kaplan M., Hayek T., Vaya J., Hoffman A., Aviram M. 2000. Oxidized monocyte-derived macrophages in aortic atherosclerotic lesion from apolipoprotein E-deficient mice and from human carotid artery contain lipid peroxides and oxysterols. Biochemical and Biophysical Research Communications. March 24;269(3):775-80.
119. Rifici V. C. 2002. Graduate faculty research: current projects. http://nutrition.rutgers.edu/faculty/rifici.htm
120. Aviram M. and Fuhrman B. 1998. Polyphenolic flavonoids inhibit macrophage-mediated oxidation of LDL and attenuate atherogenesis. Atherosclerosis. 137 Suppl:S45-50.
121. Aviram M and Fuhrman B. 1998. LDL oxidation by arterial wall macrophages depends on the oxidative status in the lipoprotein and in the cells: role of prooxidants vs. antioxidants. Molecular and Cellular Biochemistry. November;188(1-2):149-59.
122. Aviram M., Hardak E., Vaya J., Mahmood S., Milo S., Hoffman A., Billicke S.,

Draganov D., Rosenblat M. 2000. Human serum paraoxonases (PON1) Q and R selectively decrease lipid peroxides in human coronary and carotid atherosclerotic lesions: PON1 esterase and peroxidase-like activities. Circulation. May 30;101(21):2510-7.

123. ATSN (American Technion Society News). 1998. Obscure enzyme may play major role in heart disease. American Society for Technion – Israel Institute of Technology. April 9.

124. Aviram, M., Dornfeld, L., Rosenblat M., Volkova N., Kaplan M., Coleman R., Hayek T., Presser D., Fuhrman B. 2000. Pomegranate juice consumption reduces oxidative stress, atherogenic modifications to LDL, and platelet aggregation: studies in humans and in atherosclerotic apolipoprotein E-deficient mice. American Journal of Clinical Nutrition. May;71(6):1062-76.

125. Kaplan M., Hayek T., Raz A., Coleman R., Dornfeld L., Faya J., Aviram M. 2001. Pomegranate juice supplementation to atherosclerotic mice reduces macrophage lipid peroxidation, cellular cholesterol accumulation and development of atherosclerosis. Journal of Nutrition. Aug;131(8):2082-2089.

126. ATSN (American Technion Society News). 2000. Why pomegranates are better than red wine. American Society for Technion – Israel Institute of Technology. May 4.

127. Chobanian A. V., Bakris G. L., Black H. R., Cushman W. C., Green L. A., Izzo J. L., Jones D. W., Materson B. J., Oparil S., Wright J. T., Roccella E. J., and the National High Blood Pressure Education Program Coordinating Committee. 2003. The seventh report of the Joint committee on prevention, detection, evaluation, and treatment of high blood pressure. The Journal of the American Medical Association. May 14. Early Release Article.

128. CDC (Centers for Disease Control and Prevention). 2002. Hypertension. http://www.cdc.gov/nchs/fastats/hyprtens.htm

129. CDC (Centers for Disease Control and Prevention). 2002. Physician visits reach 824 million in 2000: More cardiovascular-renal, hormone and metabolic/nutrient drug visits. http://www.cdc.gov/nchs/releases/02news/physicians.htm

130. Ross R. 1999. Atherosclerosis – an inflammatory disease. New England Journal of Medicine. January14;340(2):115-26.

131. Xu C., Zarins C. K., Pannaraj P. S., Bassiouny H. S., Glagov S. 2000. Hypercholesterolemia superimposed by experimental hypertension induces differential distribution of collagen and elastin. Arteriosclerosis, Thrombosis, and Vascular Biology. 20:2566-72.

132. Mayo (Mayo Clinic.com). 2002. What is high blood pressure? http://www.mayoclinic.com/findinformation/diseasesandconditions/invoke.cfm?id=DS00100

133. AHA (American// Heart Association). 2002. Pulmonary Hypertension. http://216.185.112.5/presenter.jhtml?identifier=11076

134. Marieb E. N. 1995. In Human anatomy and physiology. Redwood City, California. The Benjamin/Cummings Publishing Company, Inc. P. 660.

135. AHA (American Heart Association). 2001. High blood pressure, what can be done. http://216.185.112.5/presenter.jhtml?identifier=4630

136. Micromedex 2001. Medlineplus Drug Information: Angiosensis-converting enzyme (Ace) inhibitors (systemic). August 18. http://www.nlm.nih.gov/medlineplus/druginfo/angiotensinconvertingenzymeace202044.html

137. Aviram M. and Dornfeld L. 2001. Pomegranate juice consumption inhibits serum angiotensin converting enzyme activity and reduces systolic blood pressure. Atherosclerosis. Sep;158(1):195-8

138. Schubert S. Y. 2001. Telephone interview of Shay Schubert, Ph.D., by the author, Shaffer Fox.

139. Schubert S. Y, Lansky E. P., Neeman I. 1999. Antioxidant and eicosanoid enzyme inhibition properties of pomegranate seed oil and fermented juice flavonoids. Journal of Ethnopharmacology. 66(1):11-7.

140. ATSN (American Technion Society News). 1999. Pomegranates may be better for you than wine, say Israeli researchers. American Society for Technion – Israel Institute of Technology. October 29.

141. Iakovleva L., Ivakhnenko A., Buniatian N. 1998. The protective action of ellagic acid in experimental myocarditis. Eksperimentalnaia Klinicheskaia Farmakologiia. May-June;61(3):32-4.

142. Ahmed S., Rahman A., Saleem M., Athar M., Sultana S. 1999. Ellagic acid ameliorates nickel induced biochemical alterations: diminution of oxidative stress. Human and Experimental Toxicology. Nov.; 18 (11):691-8.

143. ATSDR (Agency for Toxic Substances and Disease Registry). 2001. Public health statement for nickel. http://www.atsdr.cdc.gov/toxprofiles/phs15.html

144. Thresiamma K. and Kuttan R. 1996. Inhibition of liver fibrosis by ellagic acid. Indian Journal of Physiology and Pharmacology. Oct;40(4):363-6

145. ATSDR (Agency for Toxic Substances and Disease Registry). 2001. ToxFAQs for Carbon Tetrachloride. http://www.atsdr.cdc.gov/tfacts30.html

146. Cai L., and Wu C. D. 1996. Compounds from Syzygium aromaticum possessing growth inhibitory activity against oral pathogens. Journal of Natural Products. 59(10):987-90.

147. Kidd P. M. 2002. Glutathione: Systemic protectant against oxidative and free radical damage. http://www.thorne.com/altmedrev/fulltext/glut.html

148. PM (PubMed). 2002. Keyword search: Glutathione. National Center for Biotechnology Information, National Library of Medicine, National Institutes of Health. http://www.ncbi.nlm.nih.gov/entrez/query

149. Das M., Bickers D. R., Mukhtar H. 1984. Plant phenols as in vitro inhibitors of glutathione S-transferase(s). Biochemical and Biophysical Research Communications. April 30;120(2):427-33.

150. CA (Certificate of Analysis). 2001. Determination based on certificate of analysis from NBC, which includes HPLC and Folin-Denis method assays, and microbiological analysis. July 11.

151. Ramazanov Z. 2000, 2001, 2002, 2003. Telephone interviews of Zakir Ramazanov, Ph.D., by the author, Shaffer Fox.

152. CL (ConsumerLab.com). 2000. News: Pesticide contamination found in many ginseng supplements tested by ComsumerLab.com – only 9 of 22 products pass product review online today. July 11.

153. Zuin V. G. and Vilegas J. H. 2000. Pesticide residues in medicinal plants and phytomedicines. Phytotherapy Research: PTR. March;14(2):73-88.

CHAPTER 6. RHODIOLA ROSEA

1. Ramazanov Z. 1997, 1998, 2000, 2001, 2002, 2003. Telephone interviews of Zakir Ramazanov, Ph.D., by the author, Shaffer Fox.
2. Ramazanov Z. and Suarez M. 1999. In New Secrets of Effective Natural Stress and Weight Management Using Rhodiola rosea and Rhododendron caucasicum. East Cannan, CT. ATN/Safe Goods Publishing. P. 9-10.
3. IM (Intramedicine). 2001. Rhodiola. http://s-content.intramedicine.com/corpsmaples/prof-rhodiola.htm
4. Darbinyan V., Kteyan A., Panossian A., Gabriellian E., Wikman G., Wagner H. 2000. Rhodiola rosea in stress induced fatigue – a double blind cross-over study of a standardized extract SHR-5 with a repeated low-dose regimen on the mental performance of healthy physicians during night duty. Phytomedicine. 7(5):365-371.
5. TVD (The Vladivostok Daily). 2001. Extra Patrols Watching Chinese Fern Collectors. May 23
6. Underwood A. 2003. Herbal Stress Buster? Newsweek. February 3. Pp. 63-4.
7. Khaidaev Z and Menshikova T. A. 1978. In Medicinal Plants in Mongolian Medicine. Ulan-Bantor, Mongolia.
8. Magnusson B. 1992. In Beauty: herbs that touch us. Ostersund, Sweden. Berndtssons. Pp. 66-7.
9. Hoppe H. 1975. In Brogen kunde. Berlin, Germany. Walter de Gruyter. Pp. 986-7.
10. PM (PubMed). 2003. Keyword search: Rhodiola rosea. National Center for Biotechnology Information, National Library of Medicine, National Institutes of Health. http://www.ncbi.nlm.nih.gov/entrez/query
11. Brown R. P., Gerberg P. L., Ramazanov Z. 2002. Rhodiola rosea: A Phytomedicinal Overview. HerbalGram 56. http://herbalgram.org
12. Lescouflair E. 2003. Walter Bradford Cannon: Experimental Physiologist 1871-1945. http://www.harvardsquarelibrary.org/unitarians/cannon_walter.html
13. Smith M. T. 2003. Stress and Coping. Lecture #3. http://jhcourse.jhu.edu/~as200374/Stresscoping.pdf
14. Berczi I. 2003. Stress and Disease: The Contributions of Hans Selye to Neuroimmune Biology. http://home.cc.umanitoba.ca/~berczii/page4.htm
15. Tabachnik B. and Dean W. 1999. Adaptogens: Natural Protection for Stress Maladaptation and Recovery. http://www.vrp.com/art/123.asp
16. Dean W. 2003. Natural Protection and Recovery From Stress. http://www.vrp.com/art/680.asp
17. Brekhman I. I. and Dardymov I. V. 1969. New substances of plant origin which increase nonspecific resistance. Annual Review of Pharmacology. 9:419-430
18. Bolchakova I. V., Lozoskaya E. L., Sapezhinski I. I. 1996. Antioxidant properties of a series of extracts from medicinal plants. Biophysics. 42:1480-1485.
19. Salikhova R. A., Aleksandrova I. V., Mazurik V. K., Mikhailov V. F., Ushenkova L. N., Poroshenko G. G. 1997. Effect of Rhodiola rosea on the yield of mutation alterations and DNA repair in bone marrow cells. Patologicheskaia Fiziologiia i Eksperimentalnaia Terapiia. October-December, (4):22-4.
20. Razina T. G., Zueva E. P., Amosova E. N., Krylova S. G. 2000. Medicinal plant preparations used as adjuvant therapeutics in experimental oncology. Eksperimentalnaia Klinicheskaia Farmakologiia. September-October; 63(5):59-61.

21. Udintsev S. N., Krylova S. G., Fomina T. I. 1992. The enhancement of the efficacy of adriamycin by using hepatoprotectors of plant origin in metastases of Ehrlich's adenocarcinoma to the liver in mice. Oncology. 38(10):1217-22.

22. Udintsev S. N., and Shakhov V. P. 1991. The role of humoral factors of regenerating liver in the development of experimental tumors and the effect of Rhodiola rosea extract on this process. Neoplasma. 38(3):323-31.

23. Dementieva L. A., Iaremenko K. V. 1983. The study of the influence of Rhodiola rosea extract on the growth of tumors in experiment. Proceedings of Siberian Department of the USSR Academy of Science. 6:70-77.

24. Dementieva L. A., and Iaremenko K. V. 1987. Effect of Rhodiola extract on the tumor process in an experiment. Oncological Problems. 33:57-60.

25. Maslova L. V., Kondrat'ev B., Maslov L. N., Lishmanov I. B. 1994. The cardioprotective and antiadrenergic activity of an extract of Rhodiola rosea in stress. Experimental and Clinical Pharmacology. November-December;57(6):61-3.

26. Lishmanov I. B., Naumova A. V., Afanas'ev S. A., Maslov L. N. 1997. Contribution of the opioid system to realization of inotropic effects of Rhodiola rosea extracts in ischemic and reprefusion heart damage in vitro. Eksperimentalnaia Klinicheskaia Farmakologiia. May-June; 60(3):34-36.

27. Maimeshkulova L. A., Maslov L. N., Lishmanov I. B., Krasnov E. A. 1997. The participation of the mu-, delta- and kappa-opioid receptors in the realization of the anti-arrhythmia effect of Rhodiola rosea. Experimental and Clinical Pharmacopoeia. Moscow. 60:38-39.

28. Lishmanov I. B., Maslova L. V., Maslov L. N., Dan'shina E. N. 1993. The anti-arrhythmia effect of Rhodiola rosea and its possible mechanism. Biulleten Eksperimentalnoi Biologii I Meditsiny. 116(8):175-6.

29. Saratikov A., and Krasnov E. A. 1987. In Rhodiola rosea is a valuable Medicinal Plant.. Tomsk, Russia. Tomsk State University Press. Chapter VIII.

30. Ramazanov Z. 2001,2004. Data provided to the author, Shaffer Fox.

31. Kelly G. S. 2001. Rhodiola rosea: a possible plant adaptogen. Alternative Medicine Review. June;6(3):293-302.

32. Wood E. and Wood S. 1992. In The World of Psychology. Pp. 496-499. Needham Heights, Massachusetts. Allyn and Bacon, a division of Simon & Schuster.

33. Beck A. T. 1967. In Depression: Causes and treatment. Philadelphia. University of Pennsylvania Press.

34. NIMH (National Institutes of Mental Health). 2002. Depression. http://www.nimh.nih.gov/publicat/depression.cfm

35. NFDI (National Foundation for Depressive Illnesses, Inc.). 2001. www.depression.org

36. CE (Clemson Extension). 1997. Lesson 3, Understanding Depression – Yours and Theirs. Stress. HE Leaflet 68; Rep. February.

37. Ford D. E., Mead L. A., Chang P. P., Cooper-Patrick L., Wang N-Y., Klag M. J. 1998. Depression is a risk factor for coronary artery disease in men. Archives of Internal Medicine. July;158(13):1422-6.

38. Reyes-Ortiz C. A., Moreno-Macias C. H., Ceballos-Osorio J. 2001. Myocardial infarction triggered by bereavement in older women. Annals of Long-Term Care: Clinical Care and Aging. 9(7):39-43.

39. Jonas B. S. and Mussolino M. E. 2000. Symptoms of depression as a prospective risk factor for stroke. Psychosomatic Medicine. July-august;62(4):463-71.

40. Shrivastava S.and Kochar M. S. 2002. The dual risks of depression and hyperten-

sion. Postgraduate Medicine Online. June.
http://www.postgradmed.com/issues/2002/06_02/shrivastava.htm
41. Dryden J. 2001. Depression Affects Heart Rate After Heart Attack.
http://wupa.wustl.edu/record/archive/2001/03-23-01/articles/heart.html
42. Bowen R. A. 1998. Adrenal Medullary Hormones.
http://arbl.cvmbs.colostate.edu/hbooks/pathphys/endocrine/adrenal/medhormones.html
43. Green R. C., Cupples L. A., Kurz A., Auerbach S., Go R., Sadovnick D., Duara R., Kukull W. A., Chui H., Edeki T., Griffith P. A., Friedland R. P., Bachman D., Farrer L. 2003. Depression as a risk factor for Alzheimer Disease: The MIRAGE study. Archives of Neurology. May;60(5):753-9.
44. Leentjens A. F., Van Den Akker M., Metsemakers J. F., Lousberg R., Verhey F. R. 2003. Higher incidence of depression preceding the onset of Parkinson's disease: A register study. Movement Disorders. April;18(4):414-8.
45. Jorm A. F. 2000. Is depression a risk factor for dementia or cognitive decline? A review. Gerontology. July;46(4):219-227.
46. MC (Mayo Clinic). 2000. Major Depression is a Risk Factor for Seizures in Older Adults. March 9. http://www.mayoclinic.org/news2000-rst/616.html
47. Cizza G., Ravn P., Chrousos G. P., Gold P. W. 2001. Depression: a major, unrecognized risk factor for osteoporosis?.Trends in Endocrinology & Metabolism July;12(5):198-203.
48. Aldridge S. 2003. Depression Linked to Earlier Perimenopause. Health and Age. May 27. http://www.healthandage.com/Home/108!gid1=3073
49. Whitmont R. 2001. Depression and the Body.
http://www.abouttownguide.com/dutchess/articles/winter01/dpress.shtml
50. DiMatteo J. M. R., Lepper H. S., Croghan T. W. 2000. Depression is a risk factor for noncompliance with medical treatment: meta-analysis of the effects of anxiety and depression on patient adherence. Archives of Internal Medicine. July 24;160(14):2101-7.
51. Zubenko G. S., Zubenko W. N., Spiker D. G., Giles D. E., Kaplan B. B. 2001. Malignancy of recurrent, early-onset major depression: a family study. American Journal of Medical Genetics. December 8;105(8):690-9
52. Ramazanov Z. and Suarez M. 1999. In New Secrets of Effective Natural Stress and Weight Management Using Rhodiola rosea and Rhododendron caucasicum. East Cannan, CT. ATN/Safe Goods Publishing. P.39.
53. PNMH (Psych-Net Mental Health). Effects of Stress. http://www.psych-net.org/stress-effects.html
54. Bernik V. 2002. Stress:The Silent Killer. http://www.epub.org.br/cm/n03/doencas/stress_i.htm
55. Ramazanov Z. and Suarez M. 1999. In New Secrets of Effective Natural Stress and Weight Management Using Rhodiola rosea and Rhododendron caucasicum. East Cannan, CT. ATN/Safe Goods Publishing. Pp. 40-41.
56. Glaser R. and Kiecolt-Glaser J. K. 1997. Chronic stress modulates the virus-specific immune response to latent herpes simplex virus type 1. Annals of Behavioral Medicine. Spring;19(2):78-82.
57. Kiecolt-Glaser J. K., Malarkey W. B., Chee M., Newton T., Capioppo J. T., M H. Y., Glaser R. 1993. Negative behavior during marital conflict is associated with immunological down-regulation. Psychosomatic Medicine. September-October;55(5):410-2.

58. Glaser R., Kiecolt-Glaser J. K., Malarkey W. B., Sheridan J. F. 1998. The influence of psychological stress on the immune response to vaccines. Annals of the New York Academy of Sciences. May 1;840:469-55.
59. Kiecolt-Glaser J. K., Glaser R., Gravenstein S., Malarkey W. B., Sheridan J. 1996. Chronic stress alters the immune response to influenza virus vaccine in older adults. Proceedings of the National Academy of Sciences of the United States of America. April 2;93(7):3043-7.
60. Kiecolt-Glaser J. K., Page G. G., Marucha P. T., MacCallum R. C., Glaser R. 1998. Psychological influences on surgical recovery. Perspectives from psychoneuroimmunology. American Journal of Psychology. November;53(11):1209-18.
61. Marucha P. T., Kiecolt-Glaser J. K., Favagehi M. 1998. Mucosal wound healing is impaired by examination stress. Psychosomatic Medicine. May-June; 60(3): 362-5.
62. Kiecolt-Glaser J. K. and Glaser R. 1995. Psychoneuroimmunology and health consequences: data and shared mechanisms. Psychosomatic Medicine. May-June;57(3):269-74.
63. Brosschot J. F., Benschop R. J., Godaert G. L., Olff M., De Smet M., Heijnen C. J., Ballieux R. E. 1994. Influence of life stress on immunological reactivity to mild psychological stress. Psychosomatic Medicine. May-June;56(3):216-24.
64. Tortora G. and Anagnostakos N. 1990. In Principles of Anatomy and Physiology. New York: Biological Sciences Textbooks, Inc., A & P Textbooks, Inc., and Elia-Sparta, Inc., Harper Collins Publishers. Pp. 674 & 676.
65. Mayo (Mayo Clinic.com). 2000. How Stress Affects Your Health. http://www.mayoclinic.com/findinformation/conditioncenters/invoke.cfm?obj ectid=3BDDAE5C-732A-469F-87DA6683ED2A914D
66. Ross R. 1999. Atherosclerosis – an inflammatory disease. New England Journal of Medicine. January14;340(2):115-26.
67. Mayo (Mayo Clinic.com). 2002. Manage Life's Stresses. http://www.mayoclinic.com/findinformation/conditioncenters/invoke.cfm?obj ectid=B163836F-1802-4874-8281E09D35FE1076
68. Gregory M. 2001. 'Tis the Season to De-Stress and Energize. Innsbrook Today Magazine. December.
69. Kiecolt-Glaser J. K., McGuire L., robles T. F., Glaser R. 2002. Emotions, morbidity, and mortality: new perspectives from psychoneuroimmunology. Annual Review of Psychology. 53:83-107.
70. GBHF (Prevention Magazine's Giant Book of Health Facts). 1992. How the Skin Mirrors Emotions. Avenel, New Jersey. Wings Books. P. 426.
71. Fitzpatrick T. B., et al. 1979. Emotional Aspects of Cutaneous Disease. In Dermatology in General Medicine. New York. McGraw-Hill.
72. Cusimano G. S. 1978. Recognizing and Proving Damages of Traumatic Neuroses. http://www.alabamatortlaw.com/CM/Articles/doc7.pdf
73. E. I. S. (The Educational Institute of Scotland.) 2003. Preventing Stress in Higher Education: A Branch Guide. http://www.eis.org.uk/ulaStresspa.htm
74. Boeree C. The Bio-Social Theory of Neurosis. http://www.ship.edu/~cgboeree/genpsyneurosis.html
75. Friedman M. J., Charney D. S., Deutch A. Y. In Neurobiological and Clinical Consequences of Stress: From Normal Adaption to STSD. Philadelphia. Lippincott-Raven Publishers. Pp. 429-45.
76. Kaliko I. and Tarasova N. 1966. Effect of extracts of Leuzea and Golden Root on

the dynamic characteristics of the central nervous system. Tomsk: Tomsk Medical Sciences University. 1:115-120.

77. McKiernan J. M. and Lowe F. C. 1997. Side effects of Terazosin in the treatment of symptomatic benign prostatic hyperplasia. http://www.sma.org/smj97may9.htm

78. NCI (National Cancer Institute). 2002. Fatigue. http://www.meb.uni-bonn.de/cancernet/304461.html

79. FSGM (French Society of General Medicine) 2001. Depression. http://www.sfmg.org/Site%20Anglais/ang_accueilSFMG.html

80. APDST (Academic Press Dictionary of Science and Technology). 2002. Neurocirculatory asthenia. http://www.harcourt.com/dictionary/def/6/8/9/0/6890800.html

81. Tortora G. and Anagnostakos N. 1990. In Principles of Anatomy and Physiology. New York: Biological Sciences Textbooks, Inc., A & P Textbooks, Inc., and Elia-Sparta, Inc., Harper Collins Publishers. Pp. 22-23.

82. RHVPI (Random House Value Publishing, Inc.). 1996. In Webster's Encyclopedic Unabridged Dictionary of the English Language. Pp. 914, 1462, 1882.

83. MUSC (Medical University of South Carolina). 2002. The Impact of Stress on Health. http://www.musc.edu/psychiatry/slater/stress1.html

84. Holmes T. and Rahe R. 1967. The social readjustment rating scale. Journal of Psychosomatic Research. August; 11(2): 213-8.

85. RSWI (Roper Starch Worldwide, Inc.). 2001. America's Mental Health Survey 2001. The National Mental Health Association. Pp. 2, 11.

86. Nemeroff C. B. 1998. The Neurobiology of Depression. Scientific American. June.

87. Greenberg G. 2001. The Serotonin Surprise. Discover. July;22(7) Cover story. http://www.discover.com/july_01/featsurprise.html

88. Heninger G. R. 2000. Indoleamines: The Role of Serotonin in Clinical Disorders. http://www.acnp.org/G4/GN401000045/CH.html

89. Van Winkle E. 2000. The toxic mind; the biology of mental illness and violence. Medical Hypotheses. 55(4):356-368.

90. PM (PubMed). 2003. Keyword search: serotonin. National Center for Biotechnology Information, National Library of Medicine, National Institutes of Health. http://www.ncbi.nlm.nih.gov/entrez/query

91. UT (University of Texas). 2003. Neurons and Neurotransmitters: The "Brains" of the Nervous System. http://www.utexas.edu/research/asrec/neuron.html

92. Huganir R. L. 2002. Molecular Mechanisms in the Regulation of Synaptic Transmission in the Brain. http://www.hhmi.org/research/investigators/huganir.html

93. Marieb E. N. 1995. In Human anatomy and physiology. Redwood City, California. The Benjamin/Cummings Publishing Company, Inc. P. 343-362.

94. Changeux J-P. and Ricoeur P. 2000. In What Makes Us Think? A Neuroscientist and a Philosopher Argue about Human Nature, and the Brain. Princeton. Princeton University Press. P. 78.

95. SN (ScienceNet). 2003. Brain & Nervous System: Which are the Main Neurotransmitters in the Human Body? http://www.sciencenet.org.uk/database/Biology/Brain/b00375b.html

96. SRG (Serotonin Research Group). 2001. Brain's Serotonin System Declines With Age, Researchers Report. http://1-serotonin.com/serotonin-decline-with-age.html

97. SN (ScienceNet). 2003. Brain & Nervous System: How Do Anti-Depressants Work? http://www.sciencenet.org.uk/database/Biology/Brain/b00376b.html

98. Runser R. H. 1997. Antidepressants. The Grolier Multimedia Encyclopedia. Grolier Interactive, Inc.

99. Williams S. P. 1998. The serotonin transporter: a primary target for antidepressant drugs. Journal of Psychopharmacology. 12(2):1115-21

100. Ramazanov Z. and Suarez M. 1999. In New Secrets of Effective Natural Stress and Weight Management Using Rhodiola rosea and Rhododendron caucasicum. East Cannan, CT. ATN/Safe Goods Publishing. P. 42

101. Germano C. and Ramazanov Z. 1999. In Arctic Root (Rhodiola Rosea) The Powerful New Ginseng Alternative. New York. Kensington Publishing Corporation. Pp. 55, 148.

102. Krasik E. D., Petrova K., Ragulina G. 1970. Adaptogenic and stimulative effect of Rhodiola rosea extract. Proceedings of All Union Conference of Neuropathologists and Psychiatrists. Sverdlovsk. May 26-29. Pp. 215-217.

103. Krasik E., Morozova E., Petrova K., Ragulina G. G., Shemetova L. A., Shuvaeva V. P. 1970. New results on depression therapy using Rhodiola rosea extract. In Modern Problems of Psychopharmacology. Kemerovo Press Publisher. Pp. 298-300.

104. Saratikov A., Marina T., Kaliko I. 1965. Stimulative effect of Rhodiola rosea extract on brain function. Proceedings of Siberian Academy of Sciences, Biology and Medicine. 8(22):120-125.

105. Kaliko I. and Tarosova A. 1965. Effect of natural stimulants of the central nervous system. Proceedings of the 3rd Scientific Conference of Physiologists, Biochemists and Pharmacists. Tomsk; Tomsk Medical Sciences University. Pp.302-303.

106. Sudakov K. V. 1981. In Mechanisms of Emotional Stresses. Mir Publishing Press. P. 230.

107. Jorm A. F. 2001. Association of hypotension with positive and negative affect and depressive symptoms in the elderly. The British Journal of Psychiatry. 188:553-555.

108. Zaidi S. 2000. Fatigue. http:www.diabetesspecialist.com/2_thy/th01_fatigue.htm

109. Rubin R. T., Phillips J. J., McCracken J. T., Sadow T. F. 1996. Adrenal gland volume in major depression: relationship to basal and stimulated pituitary-adrenal cortical axis function. Biological Psychiatry. July 15;40(2):89-97.

110. GSDL (Great Smokies Diagnostic Laboratory). 2002. Depression and Adrenal Hormones. http://www.gsdl.com/assessments/finddisease/depression/adrenal_hormones.html

111. Merck. 2004. Adrenal Cortical Hypofunction. http://www.merck.com/mrk-shared/mmanual/section2/chapter9/9b.jps

112. Shevtsov V. A., Zholus B. I., Shervarly V. I., Vol'skij V. B., Korovin Y. P., Khristich M. P., Roslyakova N. A. Wikman G. 2003. A randomized trial of two different doses of a SHR-5 Rhodiola rosea extract versus placebo and control of capacity for mental work. Phytomedicine. March;10(2-3):95-105.

113. Zapuskalova. 1962. Russian Journal of Central Nervous System Function. 1:184-185.

114. Spasov A. A., Mandrikov V. B., Mironova I. A. 2000. The effect of the preparation rodiosin on the psychophysiological and physical adaption of students to academic load. Eksperimentalnaia Klinicheskaia Farmakologiia. 63(1):76-8.

115. Spasov A. A., Wikman G. K., Mandrikov V. B., Mironova I. A., Neumoin V. V. 2000. A double-blind, placebo-controlled pilot study of the stimulating and adaptogenic effect of Rhodiola rosea SHR-5 extract on the fatigue of students caused by stress during an examination period with a repeated low-dose regimen. Phytomedicine. April;7(2):85-9.

116. Tortora G. and Anagnostakos N. 1990. In Principles of Anatomy and Physiology. New York: Biological Sciences Textbooks, Inc., A & P Textbooks, Inc., and Elia-Sparta, Inc., Harper Collins Publishers. Pp. 798-803

117. Sal'nik. 1979. Ph.D. Thesis. Tomsk State Medicinal Sciences University.

118. Seifulla. 1999. In Sport Pharmacology Manual. Department of Medico-Biological Problems at the Russian Institute for Highest Sports Achievements, National Research Institute of Physical Culture and Sport of Russian Federation. VNIIFK - Moscow, Russia.

119. Ramazanov Z. and Suarez M. 1999. In New Secrets of Effective Natural Stress and Weight Management Using Rhodiola rosea and Rhododendron caucasicum. East Cannan, CT. ATN/Safe Goods Publishing. Pp. 35, 36.

120. Balakrishnan S. and Anuradha V. 1998. Exercise, depletion of antioxidants and antioxidant manipulation. Cell Biochemistry and Function. December;16(4):269-75.

121. Anuradha C. and Balakrishnan S. 1998. Increased lipoprotein susceptibility to oxidation following long distance running in trained subjects. Clinica Chimica Acta; International Journal of Clinical Chemistry. March;271(1):97-103

122. Anuradha C. and Balakrishnan S. 1998. Effect of training on lipid peroxidation, thiol status and antioxidant enzymes in tissues of rats. Indian Journal of Physiology and Pharmacology. January;42(1):64-70.

122. Sastre J., Asensi M., Gasco E., Pallardo F., Ferrero J., Furuka T., Vina J. 1992. Exhaustive physical exercise causes oxidation of glutathione status in blood: prevention by antioxidant administration. American Journal of Physiology. November;263(5 Pt 2):R992-5.

123. Evans W. J. 2000. Vitamin E, vitamin C, and exercise. American Journal of Clinical Nutrition. August;72(2 Suppl):647S-52S.

124. Goldfarb A. H. 1999. Nutritional antioxidants as therapeutic and preventive modalities in exercise-induced muscle damage. Canadian Journal of Applied Physiology. June;24(3):249-66.

125. Bol'shakova I. V., Lozovskaia E. L., Sapexhinskii I. I. 1998. Antioxidant properties of a series of extracts from medicinal plants. Biofizika. March-April;43(2):186-8.

126. Tortora G. and Anagnostakos N. 1990. In Principles of Anatomy and Physiology. New York: Biological Sciences Textbooks, Inc., A & P Textbooks, Inc., and Elia-Sparta, Inc., Harper Collins Publishers. Pp. 44-46.

127. NIDDK. (The National Institute of Diabetes and Digestive and Kidney Diseases). 2000. Statistics related to overweight and obesity. The National Institutes of Health. http://www.niddk.nih.gov/health/nutrit/pubs/statobes.htm

128. Chapus C., Rovery M., Sarda L., Verger R. 1988. Minireview of pancreatic lipase and colipase. Biochimie. 70:1223-34.

129. Carey M. C., and Hernell O. 1992. Digestion and absorption of fat. Seminars in Gastrointestinal Disease. 3:189-208.

130. Hernell O. 1999. Assessing fat absorption. Journal of Pediatrics. 135:4:407-9.

131. DeCaro A., Figarella C., Amic J., Michel R., Guy O. 1977. Human pancreatic lipase: a glycoprotein. Biochimica et Biophysica Acta. 490:411-19.
132. Brandt M. 2000. Introduction to Lipid Metabolism. http://chemsrvr2.fullerton.edu/meb/Chem423B/LectureNotes/Fatty_Acid_Br eakdown.pdf
133. Ramazanov Z. and Suarez M. 1999. In New Secrets of Effective Natural Stress and Weight Management Using Rhodiola rosea and Rhododendron caucasicum. . East Cannan, CT. ATN/Safe Goods Publishing. P. 29-32.
134. Abidoff M. 1997. Stimulative effect of Rhodiola rosea and Rhododendron caucasicum extract on fatty acid release in healthy volunteers. Clinical study for Russian Ministry of Health. Press release of clinical study. Moscow. P. 12.
135. Lundberg U. 1999. Catecholamines and Environmental Stress. http://www.macses.ucsf.edu/Research/Allostatic/notebook/catecholamine.html
136. Bhat N. 2003. Sudden Death and "Heart Burn." http://heartsaver.com/faq/heart1a.html
137. Tortora G. and Anagnostakos N. 1990. In Principles of Anatomy and Physiology. New York: Biological Sciences Textbooks, Inc., A & P Textbooks, Inc., and Elia-Sparta, Inc., Harper Collins Publishers. P. 600
138. Marieb E. N. 1995. In Human anatomy and physiology. Redwood City, California. The Benjamin/Cummings Publishing Company, Inc. P. 627-637.
139. Bowen R. A. 1998. Adrenal Medullary Hormones. http://arbl.cvmbs.colostate.edu/hbooks/pathphys/endocrine/adrenal/medhormones.html
140. Lishmanov Iu. B., Trifonova Zh. V., Tsibin A. N., Maslova L. V., Dement'eve L. A. 1987. Plasma beta-endorphin and stress hormones in stress adaption. 1987. Biulleten Eksperimentalnoi Biologii I Meditsiny. April;103(4):422-4.
141. Bowen R. A. 1998. Adrenal Medullary Hormones. http://arbl.cvmbs.colostate.edu/hbooks/pathphys/endocrine/adrenal/medhormones.html
142. UM (University of Miami). 2003. Cyclic AMP and Its Action. http://fig.cox.miami.edu/~1farmer/BIL265/CAMP.HTM
143. Ramazanov Z. and Suarez M. 1999. In New Secrets of Effective Natural Stress and Weight Management Using Rhodiola rosea and Rhododendron caucasicum. East Cannan, CT. ATN/Safe Goods Publishing. P. 60-61.
144. Oleynichenko V. F. 1966. Effect of Eleutherococcus and Rhodiola rosea (Golden Root) on hearing of employees of Tomsk electrochemical factory and pilots at Tomsk International Airport. In Natural Stimulators of Central Nervous System. Tomsk. Pp. 124-127.
145. TWCC (Texas Workers' Compensation Commission). 1998, 2003. Hearing Conservation. Workers' Health & Safety Division. Pub# Hs98-120B(5-03).
146. ACS (American Cancer Society). 2002. Cancer Facts & Figures 2002. http://www.cancer.org/downloads/STT/Cancerpercent20Factspercent20&percent20Figurespercent202002percent20RevCovP6P7TmPWSecured.pdf
147. MHCS (Methodist Health Care System). 2002. Cancer. http://www.methodisthealth.com/cancer/index.htm
148. Rich W. M. 2002. What is cancer? http://www.gyncancer.com/what-is.html
149. O'Connell D. 2002. Telephone interview of Daniel O'Connell, Ph.D., by the author, Shaffer Fox, for the purpose of a third party accuracy review of the paragraph cited. June 24.

150. Pitot H. C. 1997. Cancer (disease). The Grolier Multimedia Encyclopedia. Grolier Interactive, Inc.
151. Morowitz H. 1997. Cell. The Grolier Multimedia Encyclopedia. Grolier Interactive, Inc.
152. Festa F., Aglitti T., Duranti G., Ricordy R., Perticone P., Cozzi R. 2001. Strong antioxidant activity of ellagic acid in mammalian cells in vitro revealed by the comet assay. Anticancer Research. November - December;21(6A):3903-8.
153. Medem (Medem, Inc.). 2000. Cancer basics: What is cancer? http://www.medem.com/MedLB/article_detaillb.cfm?article_ID=zzzz6I0LZ6 C&sub_cat=260
154. Tortora G. and Anagnostakos N. 1990. In Principles of Anatomy and Physiology. New York: Biological Sciences Textbooks, Inc., A & P Textbooks, Inc., and Elia-Sparta, Inc., Harper Collins Publishers. P. 83-86
155. Iaremii I. N. and Grigor'eva N. F. 2002. Hepatoprotective properties of liquid extract of Rhodiola rosea. Eksperimentalnaia Klinicheskaia Farmakologiia. November-December;65(6):57-9.
156. Bocharova O. A., Matveev B. P., Baryshnikov A. I., Figurin K. M., Serebriakova R. V., Bodrova N. B. 1995. The effect of Rhodiola rosea extract on the incidence of recurrences of a superficial bladder cancer (experimental clinical research). Urologiia I Nefrologiia. March-April;(2):46-7.
157. Tortora G. and Anagnostakos N. 1990. In Principles of Anatomy and Physiology. New York: Biological Sciences Textbooks, Inc., A & P Textbooks, Inc., and Elia-Sparta, Inc., Harper Collins Publishers. P. 920.
158. Ramazanov Z. and Suarez M. 1999. In New Secrets of Effective Natural Stress and Weight Management Using Rhodiola rosea and Rhododendron caucasicum. East Cannan, CT. ATN/Safe Goods Publishing. P. 56-57.
159. Cherdinzev S. 1971. Doctoral Thesis. Uzbekistan Academy of Sciences. Tashkent, U. S. S. R.
160. Saratikov A., and Krasnov E. A. 1987. In Rhodiola rosea is a valuable Medicinal Plant. Tomsk, Russia. Tomsk State University Press. Pp. 216-27.
161. Saratikov A., and Krasnov E. A. 1987. In Rhodiola rosea is a valuable Medicinal Plant.. Tomsk, Russia. Tomsk State University Press. Pp. 69-90
162. NLM (National Library of Medicine). 2003. 17-ketosteroids. Medlineplus Medical Encyclopedia. http://www.nlm.nih.gov/medlineplus/ency/article/003460.htm
163. Kurkin V. A. and Zapesochnaya G. G. 1985. Chemical composition and pharmacological characteristics of Rhodiola rosea. Journal of Medicinal Plants, Russian Academy of Science – Moscow. 1231-45.
164. Dubichev A. G., Kurkin B. A. Zapesochnaya G. G., Vornotzov E. D. 1991. Study of Rhodiola rosea root chemical composition using HPLC. Cemico-Parmaceutical Journal. 2:188-93.
165. Ganzera M., Yayla Y., Khan I. 2001. Analysis of the marker compounds of Rhodiola rosea L. (golden root) by reversed phase high performance liquid chromatography. Chemical & Pharmaceutical Bulletin. 49(4):465-467.
166. RFMHMI (The Russian Federation Ministry of Health and Medical Industry.) 1989. Russian National Pharmacopoeia.

CHAPTER 7: CONCLUSION

1. AFC (Alliance For Children). 2002. Russia Program.
   http://www.allforchildren.org/russia.html
2. EPBP (Ethical Performance Best Practice). 2002. Nestle: Raising Health Awareness.
   http://www.ethicalperformance.com/best_practice/0202/case_studies/nestle.h
   tml
3. Ramazanov Z. 1997. Telephone interviews of Zakir Ramazanov, Ph.D., by the
   author, Shaffer Fox.
4. NCPA (National Center for Policy Information). 2001. Health Issues. Politics and
   pharmaceuticals. http://www.ncpa.org/pi/health/pd090600f.html
5. Samuelson R. J. 2000. Beware of a Regulatory Overdose. Washington Post.
   September 5. http://www.washingtonpost.com/ac2/wp-dyn?pagename=arti-
   cle&node=&contentId=A12428-2000Sep4&notFound=true
6. Rosenberg P. D. 1997. Patent. The Grolier Multimedia Encyclopedia. Grolier
   Interactive, Inc.

APPENDIX A

1. Brown R. P., Gerbarg P. L., Ramazanov Z. 2002. Rhodiola rosea: A Phytomedicinal
   Overview. HerbalGram 56. http://herbalgram.org

Index